HERBERT M. SHEL

The Complete Book for Combining Foods

How to combine foods for optimal health

This ebook was created with StreetLib Write

https://writeapp.io

Table of contents

Preface 5

Introduction 9

Chapter 1 - Classification of foodstuffs 15

Chapter 2 - Food digestion 19

Chapter 3 - Right and wrong combinations 25

Chapter 4 - Normal digestion 37

Chapter 5 - How to Combine Protein... for dinner 43

Chapter 6 - How to combine starches... for lunch 55

Chapter 7 - How to eat fruit... for breakfast 61

Chapter 8 - A salad a day 67

Chapter 9 - Dietary pattern for a week 73

Chapter 10 - How to cure indigestion 77

APPENDIX 87

Feeding raw foods 89

Protein (Important, but be cautious) 93

Gluttony and overeating 95

Eat only two meals a day 99

Dietary rules (summary) 101

Chew your food (chew, chew and chew) 105

Forget the salt 107

Pure water 109

Don't drink during meals 113
What to expect from dietary improvement 115

Original title: Food Combining Made Easy
By Herbert M. Shelton (1951)

Edition 2021 by ©David De Angelis
All rights reserved

THE EASY COMBINATION OF FOODS
of
DR. HERBERT M. SHELTON
1951

Learn what you like and eat what you enjoy appropriately.

You will love this book and rejoice in good health after you have restored your body to its natural state.

Rejoice in life, rejoice in your friendships and especially in your family. Health will make all this possible, and it will only come from a healthy diet and a natural way of life.

You will not have to start this eating program slowly but simply dive into it. Prove to your body that you are in control and that you will treat it well from this point on. Remember that losing some battles with your appetite is not as important as winning the war against disease.

Feeding oneself properly is not the private property of a religion as even an atheist can have a healthy body.

By all means, truth is where you find it, and the truth I have revealed in this book certainly did not arise with me. Truth is eternal and cannot be created or destroyed, but the lives of those who seek it can be helped while the lives of those who reject and ignore it can be destroyed.

What we really cover in this book is the utilization of the foods that Nature has given us in an effort to keep our bodies healthy. You have been given free choice. You can choose the appropriate foods to introduce into your body or you can collapse through the inappropriate use of foods and poisons. It is solely up to you to choose your life.

PREFACE

Some people search for years for a simple way of life that brings joy and health. Being healthy and energized is enjoyable even though many people do not delve into the principles of the good life when they discover them. Only YOU can make things happen and it is only YOU who will receive full benefits from appropriate choices. If you don't choose to be healthy you don't have to complain when your illness becomes your destiny.

Some people don't like making decisions. **The difficulty is not in KNOWING what is right, but in DOING what is right.** It seems difficult to overpower the habits and appetites that have formed within a certain amount of time, but what a sense of well-being when we can overcome a bad habit or start a good one!

When we change for the better, even our best friends wonder <<what's wrong>> with us. They may wonder about our good intentions especially if a good habit of ours contradicts a bad one that is practiced. People like to be in contradiction with others and are jealous if you leave them to their own devices with their bad habits. **Expect to be criticized** for your good intentions. The most perfect man of all did not have many followers, and most people voted for him to be hung on a cross. The pioneers of our country tried to create a republic instead of a democracy because they knew that the majority was not always loyal. Therefore, don't be afraid to fight for the great principles you will read about in the next few pages.

Few people believe in a functioning health system. A HEALTH SYSTEM is not necessarily the best health system. A true health system prevents diseases from happening and therefore you can avoid the present medical system that tends to cure rather than prevent. When millions of people discover this basic health system you will once again see a revival of this country.

PHYSIOLOGICAL HEALTH FACTORS can be harmful or healthy factors. The state of your health may depend on how you can completely eliminate the negative and accentuate the positive.

If you have the ability to read... you have the ability to act and change your life from this moment until death. Your willpower and determination will decide whether or not you should reach the goal of a joyful and healthy life.

Many people kid themselves when they think they're happy with a cigarette between their lips. Others are happy with a snort of cocaine. But how many alcoholics do you know who are not happy while drinking! How many fat people do you know who are happily sitting down to a banana milkshake with ice cream and cream? **The false happiness they experience will soon be replaced by one of the many illnesses or health problems they can only imagine.** To compensate for their problems they are probably stuffing their faces with aspirin, sleeping pills, antacids, tranquilizers, etc.

We can be content by controlling our appetites and developing positive living habits. It will certainly take some time to corrupt willpower and abandon a bad habit, but it only takes a little willpower to start a new habit. A healthier and happier life depends on many positive physiological factors affecting the body and mind.

The purpose of this book is not to "know it all and say it all." By paying attention to the positive factors you will be able to achieve goals or by paying attention to the negative factors you will be able to eliminate them.

This book could have a major turning point in your life. Many people will praise it, others will condemn it, but condemnations will not change the truths you will find written here. Ignoring the truth means suffering the consequences of a past life and continuing to live with wrong appetites and poor habits. The choice is yours. You have been given freedom of choice. How you will use that freedom is your business alone.

What are you doing for your children's bodies by ignoring physiological factors? Do they have colds, headaches, and stomachaches? Are they tired, listless, hyperactive, or sick?

We do not intend to cure these diseases. Cure is not the subject of this book. **There can be no disease if there is no cause, so it is necessary to eliminate the cause. It is** a very simple premise. If there is no cause for a headache you will not suffer it. If there is no cause for vomiting you will not vomit. If there is no cause for a fever there will be no fever. **All of these so-called ailments are almost all natural ways in which the body gets rid of something wrong that we put into it. For example: when we sweat, the sweat glands get rid of salt which is a poison to the body.** Some doctors and nutritionists still believe that the body needs a certain form of salt called sodium chloride. Our habits have taught us to take pleasure in the taste of salt. The body can process all the amount of salt it needs from the natural foods we eat. A couple of tablespoons full of salt will be able to make you sick and in case kill you if you want.

I hope that this book will be just the beginning of a great adventure in life.

INTRODUCTION

A few years ago I was at a friend's house with whom, along with other people present, we were watching a television programme. One of the commercials featured a breakfast bowl into which a man poured a popular cereal product. To this he added two full tablespoons of white sugar. He then topped it with a sliced banana and a handful of raisins. To the mixture he had created he added, last, cream and milk in large quantities. As he showed the preparation of the dish, he used a variety of words to convince the listening public that his dish was both tasty and nutritious. When he had finished, one of the women in the group exclaimed: <<Every time I eat a dish like that, I get heartburn!>>. I replied: <<This happens to you and to several million other people.>> No human digestive system, in fact, is suited to digest a meal like that.

In nature, no animal ever eats a mixture of such disparate products. It is surely not a matter for human intelligence that, day after day, millions of men, women and children continue to consume such dishes and to stuff themselves with medicines in an attempt to alleviate the ailments they cause.

Every year millions of dollars are spent on digestives or similar products just to soothe the gastric difficulty that is almost inevitable after such a meal. Among the most famous, containing almost all sodium carbonate, we remember: Alka-Seltzer, Diger-Seltz, **Digestivo Antonetto**, etc. Many persons, then, resort to the ancient habit of using bicarbonate of soda; others use Milk of Magnesia. These drugs, which alone appear harmful, provide only temporary relief to the troubles caused by indigestion.

Despite the unnecessary suffering that millions of people experience on a daily basis and the considerable sums of money they spend in search of relief, there are unfortunately still many who, even for their own good, do not make the effort to feed themselves properly.

There is an old proverb that says: <<Actions, not words, are what count>>. The way we present the combinations of foods is such that it allows the common man to prepare his own food program. It has no need of expensive scientific verifications: everyone can organize his own meals in an ideal combination, following the rules contained in this book and then verify the results. Results that can then be compared with those obtained from the previous diet.

Not too long ago one of my representatives received a letter from a woman in Pennsylvania, to whom he had sold a copy of "The Easy Combination of Foods." I quote parts of it here: <<Writing letters of flattery is not my style, but this one has a deeper meaning. It is a letter of appreciation and thanks. A fortunate day was when I received your literature and requested a copy of The Easy Combination of Foods, by Herbert M. Shelton.>>

<<**For years and years I had suffered from indigestion, gas in the stomach, bloating and pain**. Now that I try to combine foods in the right way, the indigestion and discomfort have disappeared. No more gas, bloating, Alka-Seltzer or bicarbonate.>>

<<Why don't people make use of this simple method? Surely because they don't know it.>>

I have received many letters like this. Many people have talked to me personally and confirmed the same concept. **Many people say they feel relief from the first time they eat a meal that is ideally combined**. Just recently a man told me how he and his family got rid of digestive problems by eating foods that were combined in the right way. He and his family also found they could survive without the need for medication. Many other people have told me how, by combining foods, they were able to end certain allergies.

The human digestive system, according to nature, is not designed to digest elaborate meals. Seven-course or twenty-one-course meals were not planned by nature when it created man's digestive system. The person who sits in front of a table laden with all kinds of foods and eats everything, "from appetizer to dessert," will surely suffer from indigestion. If eating complicated meals becomes a habit, neglecting one's enzymatic limits, intestinal disorders will become chronic. Wherever he goes, he will have to take his supply of medicines with him. In fact, the habit of carrying pills in one's pocket, is strongly encouraged by practitioners. It seems more important to have an artificial remedy available than to learn to eat in such a way as to avoid the need for medication. It seems more important to enrich the pharmaceutical companies than to protect one's own health.

Because this book has been prepared for everyone and not just vegetarians, the menus presented contain mixed meals and meals for vegetarians only. This is not a compromise or a tacit defection from vegetarianism: it is just a way to meet the different needs of the various classes of readers.

Both on the medical side and on the part of the advocates of the so-called healing schools and of allopathy, objections have been raised to the avoidance of certain food combinations and the consumption of others. These objections, are based on the belief that the stomach of man is adapted to digest all kinds of food combinations. I shall not linger long in countering these objections, for the arguments presented in the book are in themselves an answer.

More than sixty years' work in the field of nutrition, concerned with young and old, healthy and sick, rich and poor, educated and ignorant, and more than fifty years spent in institutional practice, give me a certain degree of authority in the matter. I have devoted more than sixty years to the study of dietetics, directing my attention to the care and feeding of many thousands of people. An intelligent reader should understand that so vast an experience qualifies me best to set forth the subjects which form the text of this publication, bearing in mind the circumstance that it has not been time spent in administering medicine to patients. **Few physicians study dietetics, and even fewer apply it in the treatment of their patients. Their most common suggestion is: <<eat whatever you wish>>**.

This book is not intended to assert that any dietary program or combination of foods can cure disease. I do not believe in cures, but I do believe, and I am prepared to prove it, that in all cases of disease, where the organic damage does not appear too serious to impair recovery, the removal of the causes enables the vital forces and processes, together with the normal materials of life, to restore health and wholeness. Food, indeed, is but one of the materials of life.

As an essential basis, the work of a hygienist must ensure that the individual receives the benefit of all hygienic means in their fullness because, only in this way, can he have a chance to recover. An **attentive reader should have no difficulty in understanding that hygienic cures are the only rational and radical cures that in any age and in any part of the world have been administered to**

the sick. There will come a time when all forms of disease will be "treated" on the basis of infallible hygienic principles. When sound principles exist, they can be applied not to just one or two diseases, but to all. The same basic principles will underlie every kind of disease. Even in cases where surgery is to be used, the rules of hygiene should always be used to prepare the field for surgery.

Why worry about the combination of foods? Why not mix them confusedly and eat them roughly? Why waste time on such matters? Perhaps animals follow rules when combining foods?

The answers to these questions are simple. Let's start with the last one. Animals eat very simply without having to worry too much about combinations. What is certain, however, is that carnivorous animals, along with protein, do not consume carbohydrates. They do not eat acids along with protein. The deer, which grazes in the forest, combines its foods very little. The squirrel, which eats nuts, will probably, along with these, not consume any other food. It has been observed that birds eat insects and seeds at separate times. In nature, no animal, has at its disposal the great variety of foods which is characteristic of civilized man. Primitive man certainly did not have a wide choice of food. He, like the animals, fed himself in a very simple way.

As we will see later, the digestive enzymes in the human digestive tract have well-defined limits, and when, by eating disproportionately, you exceed these limits, you run into digestive problems. The right combination of foods is the healthiest way to respect enzyme limitations. Combine foods appropriately, do not eat unreasonably, and digestion will appear better and certainly more regular.

Food that is not digested has no value. Eating and then letting food "spoil" in the stomach means not only wasting it but also something more serious: food that decomposes in the stomach produces poisons that are harmful to the body. The right combination of foods, therefore, not only ensures better nutrition, as a result of better functioning digestion, but also serves to protect against poisoning.

A surprising number of food allergies disappear completely when individuals who are considered allergic, learn how to feed themselves, combining foods in such a way that they can be digested.

Their problem is not allergy, but indigestion. **Allergy is the term given to protein poisoning.** Indigestion gives, as a result, decay poisoning, also a protein poisoning. Normal digestion produces nutrients; not poisons to be put into the blood stream.

Well-digested proteins are not poisonous substances.

With my vast experience behind me, I offer this book to the most attentive readers, in the hope that they will use the information it contains in the best possible way, establishing better health and living, therefore, longer. To those who still have doubts, I can only say: <<Read this book and convince yourself of its importance>>. Judging without knowing, in fact, means putting an end to knowledge. Do not limit your horizons and do not deprive yourself of the opportunity to improve your health by condemning, without reason, the simple rules presented in this book.

CHAPTER 1 - CLASSIFICATION OF FOODSTUFFS

Foods are those substances which, through the complex processes of digestion, are processed by the body and assimilated by the blood. **Useless substances, such as medicines, are poisonous.** To be useful, the substance must not contain harmful and unnecessary ingredients.

Tobacco, for example, which is a plant, contains protein, carbohydrates, minerals, vitamins and water. For this reason, it should be considered a food. But, in addition to these elements, it contains considerable quantities of poisons, including some of the most dangerous existing in nature. Tobacco, therefore, is not a food.

Foodstuffs, as they come to us from the garden, or from the shop, are made up of water and organic compounds such as proteins, carbohydrates (sugars, starches, pentosans), fats (oils), mineral salts and vitamins. Generally, they also contain more or less variable amounts of useless materials.

Foods, the essential materials of nutrition, vary enormously in character and quality. Therefore, for convenience, we have classified them according to their composition and origin. The following classifications will serve the reader as a guide in combinations.

PROTEINS

Protein foods are those that contain a high percentage of protein. The most important ones are as follows:

Walnuts, Soy, Olive, Cereals, Peanuts, Avocado, Dried beans, Meat (except fat), Milk, Dried peas, Cheese,

AMIDS

Carbohydrates are starches and sugars. In the following classification they have been divided into three distinct groups: starches, sugars (including syrups)

and sweet fruits.

AMIDS
Cereals, Dried beans (except soya beans), Dried peas, Potatoes, Chestnuts, Peanuts, Winter melon, Banana, Pumpkin, Caladium roots, Topinamburi (Tuberous sunflower),

SUGARS
Dark sugar, White sugar, Powdered sugar, Maple Syrup, Cane syrup, Honey,

SWEET FRUIT
Banana, Dates, Figs, Raisins, Moscato, Plums , Khaki, Mango, Papaya, Cherries, Dried pears

SLIGHTLY STARCHY
Cauliflower, Beets, Carrots Cherries, Saxifrage,

FATS

Fats also include oils, as follows:

Olive oil, Butter, Fatty meats, Soya oil, Cream, Cottonseed oil, Sunflower seed oil, Nocelline oil, Avocado, Sesame oil, Corn oil, Butter substitutes, Tallow (solid vegetable fat), American walnut, Walnuts in general,

ACID FRUIT

Most of the acids we ingest as food are represented by acidic fruits. The main types are as follows:

Orange, Tomato, Sour grapes, Grapefruit, Lemon, Fishing, Pineapple, Lime, Sour plums, Pomegranate, Frozen apples,

SEMI-ACID FRUIT

The semi-acid fruit is as follows:

Fresh figs, Sweet Peaches, Blueberries, Pears, Sweet apples, Sweet Plums, Sour cherries (amarasco), Apricots,

VEGETABLES

This classification includes all qualities of vegetables, without reference to colour or anything else. The main ones are:

Lettuce, Primrose, Rhubarb, Celery, Chinese cabbage, Watercress, Endive, Garlic onion, Onion, Chicory, Mustard, Shallot, Cabbage, Romici (agri), Leek, Cauliflower, Turnip, Garlic, Broccoli, Green cabbage, Zucchini, Brussels sprouts, Verbasco, Scarola, Turnip rape, Rapeseed, Beets (green), Spinach, Green corn, Turnip greens, Thistles, Eggplants, Bamboo shoots, Hibiscus, Carduccio, Broccoli, Cucumber, Radish, Sweet peppers, Sorrel, Parsley, Asparagus, Shower head,

MELONI

Watermelon, "Casaba", Persian, Winter melon, Cantalupo, Netting, Nutmeg, Long,

CHAPTER 2 - FOOD DIGESTION

As already stated, food constitutes the raw material of nutrition, since it is composed of proteins, carbohydrates, and fats, and cannot be used directly by the body, but must first undergo a process of disintegration and refining (in truth a series of processes), known as digestion. Although the digestive process is partly mechanical, as in the chewing and swallowing of food, the physiology of digestion is, in large part, the study of the chemical changes that food undergoes as it passes through the alimentary canal. We will focus more of our attention on digestion in the mouth and stomach, rather than digestion in the intestines.

The changes which food undergoes in the digestive process are effected by a group of agents which take the name of **enzymes** or ferments. Owing to the fact that the conditions under which they come into action are well defined, it becomes necessary to pay close attention to the simple rules which underlie the proper combination of foods; rules which, by the way, have been determined according to the chemistry of digestion. The long and patient efforts of many physiologists, in the most disparate parts of the world, have brought to light the enzymatic limitations; unfortunately, however, these same physiologists have overlooked their importance, and have created a series of fictitious reasons to justify the poor eating habits of modern man. They have avoided at all events putting into practice the vital discoveries which are the result of their meticulous research study. Natural Hygienists do not act in this way. We try to organize the rules of life on the principles of biology and physiology.

Before going on to study the enzymes of the mouth and stomach, let us try to frame them in a general sense. An enzyme may be defined as a catalyst of a physiological nature. Studying chemistry, it was soon discovered that many substances that did not combine with each other could do so if they were put in contact with a third substance. This third substance did not interfere in any way in the combination or in the reaction, but its presence seemed to cause both. This agent or substance came to be called the catalyst - the process, catalysis.

Plants and animals produce soluble catalytic substances, colloidal in nature and resistant to heat, which they use in the various processes of division of compounds and in their manufacture. These substances have been called enzymes: many are known, and almost all of them are of a proteinic character. Those with which we shall be concerned are the digestive enzymes. These reduce the complex substances of food into simpler compounds suitable for introduction into the blood stream and for use by the cells of the body in the production of new cells.

Since the action of enzymes in the digestion of food is reminiscent of fermentation, these substances were initially classified as ferments. Fermentation, however, is carried out by means of organized ferments: bacteria. The products of fermentation are not identical to those of the enzymatic disintegration of food and do not constitute nutritional substances. Instead, they are poisonous. Decomposition (putrefaction) also results in the formation of poisons instead of nutrients.

Each enzyme has a specific action. That is, it acts only on one type of food substance. Enzymes that act on carbohydrates cannot also have an effect on proteins or salts or fats. The specificity is even more particular: for example, in the digestion of closely related substances, such as disaccharides (complex sugars), the enzyme that acts on maltose cannot also have an effect on lactose. Each sugar requires its own specific enzyme. The physiologist Howell argues that, each enzyme, can produce more than one type of ferment action.

This specific action of enzymes is very important because in the digestion of food there are several stages, each requiring the action of a different enzyme. In turn, each enzyme is capable of doing its work only if the one that preceded it has done itss properly. If pepsin, for example, has not transformed the proteins into peptones, the enzymes that must transform the peptones into amino acids will not be able to act on the proteins.

The substance on which the enzyme acts is called substrate (substrate). Starch is the substrate of ptyalin. Dr. N. Philip Norman, formerly a teacher of grastroenterology at the New York Polyclinic Medicai School and Hospital in New York City, says: <<Studying the actions of enzymes, one is struck by Emil Fisher's thought that for every lock there must be a key. If the ferment represents the lock and its substrate the key, and if the key does not fit perfectly into

the lock, a reaction cannot occur. Consequently, **is it not logical to consider it injurious to the digestive cells to mix together, in the same meal, different kinds of carbohydrates, fats and proteins?** Since it is true that the same types of cells produce similar but not identical locks, it is logical to argue that such a mixture aggravates to the extreme limit the physiological functions of these cells>>. Fisher, who was a famous physiologist, maintained that the specificity of the various enzymes is related to the structure of the substance on which they act. It seems that each enzyme is suitable only for a particular structure.

Digestion begins in the mouth. Through the process of chewing, all food is broken down into smaller particles that are mixed with saliva. Of the chemical part of digestion, only the starch part begins in the mouth. Saliva, normally an alkaline liquid, contains an enzyme called ptyalin which, acting on starches, transforms them into maltose, a complex sugar, which in turn, in the intestine, is transformed into dextrose (simple sugar). The action of ptyalin on starches is preparatory as maltose cannot have an effect on starches. It appears that amylase, the enzyme of the pancreatic secretion which divides starches, acts on starch in the same way as ptyalin; that is, so that starch which escapes digestion in the mouth and stomach may be broken down into maltose and acro-dextrin; provided, of course, that it has not undergone fermentation before reaching the intestine.

In the mucous membrane of the stomach there are numerous glands that secrete gastric juice. This can give rise to a wide range of reactions, from almost neutral to strongly acidic, depending on the nature of the food consumed. It contains two enzymes: pepsin, which acts on proteins, and lipase, which acts slightly on fats. We will only deal with pepsin here. This enzyme is able to initiate the digestion of any protein; which is very important as it seems to be the only one to have this possibility.

The various enzymes which divide proteins act on the different stages of their digestion. It may happen that no enzyme can act on proteins at the stage preceding that for which it proves suitable. Erepsin, for example, present in the intestinal and pancreatic juices, cannot act on complex proteins, but only on peptides and polypeptides, reducing them to amino acids. Without the prior action of pepsin reducing proteins to peptides, erepsin would not take action. Pepsin can only act in an acidic medium and is destroyed by alkalis. Low temperatures, such as ice-cold drinks, delay or even suspend the action of pepsin. Alcohol even precipitates this enzyme.

So that the sight or smell of food may cause profuse salivation, the so-called "mouth watering", in the same way it may also cause an abundant production of gastric juice, a "stomach watering". However, the taste of food is the most important factor in the production of profuse salivation. The physiologist Carlson was not very successful in repeated attempts to induce a flow of gastric juice by making subjects chew different substances, or by stimulating the nerve endings of the mouth with other substances than food. In other words, when food, introduced into the mouth, is not digested, no secretions occur. The organism performs a selective procedure, and, as we shall see later, performs different kinds of operations according to the various species to be processed.

In his experiments on "conditioned reflexes," Pavlov noted that it is not necessary to put food in the mouth to cause a secretion of gastric juice. Just teasing the dog with tasty treats, for example, can do the trick. He even discovered that noises or other manifestations that have some connection with the moment of feeding could cause secretion.

It is necessary to devote a few brief paragraphs to an analysis of the organism's ability to adapt its secretions to the different types of food consumed. Subsequently, we shall discuss its limitations. McLeod, in his Physiology in Modern Medicine, states : <<Pavlov's observations on the responses of the gastric sacs of dogs to meat, bread and milk, are very interesting in that they prove the fact that the operation of the gastric secretory mechanism is adapted to the materials to be digested>>.

This adaptation is made possible because the gastric secretions are the result of the work of some five million microscopic glands embedded in the walls of the stomach, many of which secrete gastric juice. **The quantities and proportions of the different elements composing it make the gastric juice of a variable character and easily adapted to digest different kinds of food.** As a result of this, the gastric juice, may give rise to an almost neutral, slightly acid reaction and may contain more or less pepsin according to need. There is also the time factor: the character of the juice may appear very different in relation to the digestive stage, that is, as the food requirements are met.

Similar adaptation also occurs when saliva adjusts to different types of food and digestive needs. Light acids, for example, cause an abundant secretion of saliva, while light alkalis cause no secretion at all. Even harmful substances cause secretion of saliva, in order to eliminate harmful material. Physiologists emphasize the fact that if one has at least two different types of glands in the mouth, both of which are active, it is possible to produce a wide range of variations in the character of the secretion.

A good example of this capacity of the body to modify and adapt its secretions according to the varying needs of different kinds of food is given to us by the dog. With the administration of meat it produces, in fact, mainly from the submandibular glands, a thick and viscous secretion of saliva. With the administration of dry food (dried or freeze-dried meat) there will be a secretion, from the parotid gland, very abundant and watery. The mucous secretion produced with meat serves to lubricate the food bolus and thus facilitate swallowing. The aqueous secretion in powdered foods, serves to remove every small grain from the mouth. Therefore, it appears that the type of juice produced is determined according to the task it is to perform. As has been previously stated, ptyalin does not act on sugar. **By the consumption of sugar an abundant secretion of saliva is caused, but this does not contain ptyalin.** If starches are ingested, no saliva is produced. With meat and fats, there is no production of ptyalin. These examples of adaptation are few when compared with all that could be given. It seems probable that a greater adaptation takes place in the gastric secretion than in the salivary. Such arguments do not appear to be without value to those who are desirous of feeding themselves in such a way as to permit regular digestion, but too often physiologists tend to ignore or minimize them. In the following chapters we shall have an opportunity of dealing with these matters in great detail.

There are grounds for believing that man, like animals, once instinctively possessed the ability to avoid wrong combinations of food, and that in part this ability is still in his baggage. But, having built the empire of intellect on the ruins of instinct, man is compelled to seek, under the most surprising circumstances and amidst the most insane errors and methods, his way of life. This will happen until he has attained a degree of knowledge and comes into possession of such principles as will enable him to govern his conduct in the light of their teachings. Then, instead of ignoring the vast amount of physiological knowledge concerning the digestion of food, or neglecting it as is the habit of physiologists, man, an intelligent being, should be taught to make proper use of this knowledge. If the physiology of digestion enables one to adopt habits which improve this process, only a fool can ignore its value both in health and in disease.

CHAPTER 3 - RIGHT AND WRONG COMBINATIONS

In order to make perfectly clear what food combinations fatigue our enzyme limitations, it will be necessary to consider the combinations one at a time and then treat them in the light of the digestive processes we have discussed in the previous chapter. An intelligent reader will consider this analysis interesting and instructive.

3.1 Combinations of acids and starches

In the preceding chapter we learned that **a mild acid is capable of destroying the ptyalin of the saliva. With the destruction of the latter, the digestion of starches stops.** Physiologist Stiles says: <<If the food set appears acidic from the beginning, it is difficult to think that saliva can produce hydrolysis (enzymatic digestion of starches). Nevertheless, we continue to eat acidic fruit before our cereal breakfast without noticing any harmful effects. The starch that is not digested at this stage is then "processed" by the pancreatic juice with satisfactory end results. However, it may be intelligently deduced that the greater the work done by the saliva, the less will be the work of the other secretions and the better, most probably, will be the digestion.

Oxalic acid, diluted in quantities of 1 part in 10,000 completely arrests the action of ptyalin. In one or two tablespoonfuls of vinegar there is sufficient ethanoic acid to suspend salivary digestion altogether. The acid of tomatoes, oranges, grapefruits, lemons, limes, pineapples, green apples, unripe grapes, and other acid fruits are sufficient to destroy the ptyalin of the saliva and arrest the digestion of starches. Without apparently understanding the reasons for this, Dr. Percy Howe of Harvard, says: <<Many people who cannot eat oranges after a meal, derive, on the contrary, great benefit if they eat them fifteen or thirty minutes beforehand.>>

All physiologists agree that acids, even light acids, destroy ptyalin. Until it can be shown that saliva is capable of digesting starch without the presence of ptyalin, we must continue to insist that combinations between starches and acids are not digestible. The layman's assertion that any combination of foods can be considered right is based on ignorance and preconception. For the considerations just made **the rule should be: eat starches and acids in separate meals.**

3.2 Combinations of proteins and starches

Chitteden demonstrated that a minimum percentage of hydrochloric acid (0.003%) was sufficient to suspend the process of starch division (amylolysis), and that an increase of acidity, even if slight, interrupted the process, but destroyed the enzyme. In his Textbook of Physiology Howell, speaking of gastric lipase, asserts that:«this type of lipase is immediately destroyed in the presence of an acidity of 0.2% hydrochloric acid, so that, if it appears to be of functional importance in gastric digestion, its action, like that of ptyalin, must be confined to the initial period of digestion before the contents of the stomach have reached their normal acidity» (Italics mine).Here we will not deal with the destruction of lipase caused by the hydrochloric acid of the stomach, but with the destruction of ptyalin by the same acid.

The physiologist Stiles says: <<The acid which greatly aids gastric digestion, appears prohibitive in salivary digestion>>. Speaking of pepsin he says: <<The ability to digest proteins is manifested only by an acid reaction, and is totally absent when the measure is distinctly alkaline. The conditions which permit the peptic digestion are, therefore, those which exclude the action of the saliva>>. Of the enzyme ptyalin then, he says: <<since the enzyme is extremely sensitive to acid and the gastric juice is decidedly acid, it was thought that salivary digestion could not take place in the stomach>>. The gastric juice destroys ptyalin and, therefore, interrupts the digestion of starch. If this were true, how could the digestion of starchy foods take place?

The answer to this question is to be found in the ability of the digestive system to adapt its secretions to the digestive needs of different types of food, provided, of course, that the limits of this adaptation mechanism are respected. Dr. Richard C. Cabot of Harvard, who neither condemned nor extolled any particular method of combining foods, wrote: <<When carbohydrates are ingested, the stomach secretes a gastric juice of a different composition from that produced in the presence of proteins. This is the response of the stomach to a particular demand made upon it. It is one of the many examples of choice made by the parts of the organism, generally considered unconscious and without its own decision-making power>>. The secret is this: when the stomach ingests a starchy food, it secretes a different kind of juice from that produced in the presence of a protein food.

Pavlov showed that each kind of food causes a particular activity of the digestive glands; that the capacity of the juice varies with the quality of the food; that particular modifications of the glands are necessary according to different foods; that the strongest juice is produced only when necessary.

By ingesting bread, a small amount of hydrochloric acid is introduced into the stomach. The juice produced in the presence of bread is of almost neutral reaction. When the starch in the bread is digested, a large amount of hydrochloric acid is introduced into the stomach to facilitate the digestion of the bread protein. The two processes cannot occur efficiently at the same time. On the contrary, the secretions appear minutely programmed, both in character and in time, according to the varying needs of the food substances ingested.

Herein lies the answer for those who do not believe in the combination of foods as "nature combines various food substances in the same food." There is a great difference between the digestion of one "food," however complex its composition may be, and the digestion of a "mixture" of different foods. In the presence of a single type of food, a combination of starches and proteins, the body is able to adapt its juices, in intensity according to the digestive needs of that food, but when two foods are ingested which present different or even opposite digestive needs, this adaptation of the juices becomes impossible. If meat and bread are eaten together, instead of the production of an almost neutral juice during the first two hours of digestion, a highly acid juice will be produced and the digestion of starch will be immediately interrupted.

It should never be forgotten that physiologically, the first steps in the digestion of starches and proteins take place in opposite environmental circumstances: starches need an alkaline environment, proteins an acid one. In this connection, V. H. Mottram, professor of physiology at the University of London, in his Physiology, states that when in the stomach the food comes into contact with the gastric juice, salivary digestion cannot take place. He states, <<The gastric juice digests proteins, and the saliva, starches. It is therefore obvious, that to obtain a regular digestion, the meat (proteins) should form the first part of the meal, and the starches the second: which is often commonly the case. Meat generally precedes all kinds of desserts.>>

Mottram explains the argument in this way: <<The distal extremity of the stomach is the one in which the movement takes place that allows the food to mix with the gastric juice... But, while the food that is in the still extremity is still under the influence of the saliva, the one that is in the moving extremity comes into contact with the acid gastric juice making the action of the saliva impossible>>. In a nutshell, this means that by eating the proteins first and then the starches, the proteins will be ingested in the lower part of the stomach and the starches in the upper part.

Imagining in the stomach a line of demarcation between foods, and following your statements, it appears that people, neither instinctively nor for any other reason, consume proteins and starches in this way. Perhaps in England there is a custom of eating meat at the beginning of lunch and pudding at the end, in the same way as we consume dessert at the end of lunch, but, both there and here, there is a custom of eating starches and proteins together. When the common man eats meat, eggs, or cheese, he combines bread with protein. Hot dogs, **ham sandwiches,** hamburgers, eggs and bread, and other similar combinations of protein and starch are the most common way of consuming such foods. With a diet of this kind it happens that the proteins and starches are thoroughly mixed in both ends of the stomach.

Howell argues much the same thing: <<A point of considerable importance is to understand how much, under usual circumstances, salivary digestion has effect on starchy foods. The process of chewing in the mouth perfectly mixes the food and saliva, but the bolus is swallowed too quickly to allow the enzyme to complete its action. In the stomach the gastric juice is sufficiently acid to destroy ptyalin, and it is for this reason, therefore, that it was once thought that salivary digestion was immediately arrested by the introduction of food into the stomach, and that at any rate, as a digestive process, it possessed no great

value. At a later date, as the field of knowledge deepened, the contrary was demonstrated, namely, that part of the food consumed at an ordinary meal could remain in the bottom of the stomach for an hour or more without being in the least touched by the acid secretion. Therefore, there is every reason to believe that salivary digestion may be carried on in the stomach without too much restriction>>.

It is obvious that salivary digestion can only take place in the stomach on a small amount of food, provided, of course, that one consumes the usual harmful combinations such as bread with meat, bread with eggs, bread with cheese, bread with other proteins or potatoes with proteins. When you eat a hamburger or frankfurter sandwich, you do not eat the meat first and then the bread. They are chewed, mixed and swallowed together. The stomach does not have a mechanism that can separate these mixed substances and direct them, then, into the different cavities.

In nature, such combinations do not exist; animals tend to eat only one type, of food at a time. The carnivorous animal will certainly not combine starches with its proteins. Birds consume insects and seeds at different times during the day. Surely, even for man, this would be the best food program as, the systems suggested by Mottram would not provide good results.

Based on the physiological issues we have presented, we can formulate the second rule about food combinations: *"Eat protein foods and carbohydrate foods at separate times."*

This means that grains, breads, potatoes and other starchy foods should not be eaten along with meat, eggs, cheese, nuts and other protein foods.

3.3 Proteinand proteincombinations

Two proteins of different character and composition, joined together with other food constituents, in order to be well digested cause **changes in the digestive secretions and in the time of secretion**. For example, the strongest juice goes with milk in the last hour of digestion, and with meat in the first hour.

Do these secretion times have any value? Generally in our eating habits, there is a tendency to ignore these facts, and even physiologists are inclined to overlook them. Eggs receive the strongest secretion at a different time from meat and milk. It is logical, therefore, to say that **eggs should not be consumed at the same time as meat or milk**. It should not be forgotten how tuberculosis patients were greatly injured by the administration of eggs and milk together. **For centuries and centuries the Orthodox Jews abstained from consuming meat and milk at the same meal.**

The fact is that the digestive process is modified to meet the needs of each protein food, and for this reason, it is impossible for the modification to be such that it meets the needs of two different types of protein consumed at the same time. This does **not necessarily mean that two different types of meat or nuts cannot be eaten at the same meal; it does mean**, however, that protein combinations such as meat and eggs, meat and nuts, meat and cheese, eggs and nuts, cheese and nuts, milk and nuts, etc., should not be eaten. A single protein food will ensure greater digestive efficiency.

Our rule therefore, should be "Eat only one protein-concentrated food per meal".

The following objection has been raised to this rule: since the different proteins vary so much in their amino acid contents and the body needs adequate amounts of some of these, it seems necessary to consume more than one protein in order to ensure an adequate supply of amino acids. But, since most people consume more than one meal a day and protein is present in almost all foods, the objection no longer exists. It **is not necessary to consume all the protein you need at every meal.**

3.4 Combinations of acids and proteins

The active work of breaking down (digesting) complex protein substances into simpler ones, which takes place in the stomach and is the first step in protein digestion, is carried out by the enzyme pepsin. Pepsin acts only in an acid environment and its action is interrupted by alkali. The gastric juice can be almost neutral to strongly acidic depending on the type of food that is put into the stomach. When protein is ingested, the gastric juice is acidic, as it must provide a favorable environment for the action of pepsin.

Since pepsin is only active in an acidic environment, it was erroneously assumed that ingesting acids during a meal would facilitate protein digestion. In truth, on the contrary, these acids inhibit the diffusion of gastric juice and thus interfere in the digestion of proteins. Medicines and **acid fruits ruin gastric digestion, either by the destruction of pepsin or by the inhibition of that secretion. In the presence of acid in the mouth and stomach, gastric juice is not emitted.** The famous Russian physiologist, Pavlov, successfully demonstrated the injurious effect of acids on digestion: whether derived from acid fruit, or from the acid elements resulting from fermentation. Acid fruit, by inhibiting the emission of gastric juice-which is needed in abundance for the digestion of proteins-seriously injures such digestion and causes putrefaction.

A normal stomach secretes the acid necessary for pepsin to digest a normal amount of protein. An abnormal stomach may secrete too much acid (hyperacidity) or too little (hypoacidity). In either case, however, consuming protein and acid together does nothing to aid digestion. While pepsin is not active except in the presence of hydrochloric acid (no other type of acid has been found to activate this enzyme), excess gastric acidity prevents its action. Acid in excess destroys pepsin.

Based on these simple facts of the physiology of digestion, we formulate our rule: *"Eat protein and acid in separate meals."*

If we consider the actual process of protein digestion in the stomach and the inhibitory effects of acids on gastric secretion, we immediately realize the error contained in the habit of consuming pineapple juice, or grapefruit or tomato juice with meat, or of "beating" eggs together with orange juice to form the famous "pepcocktail" advertised by some other pseudo-dietologists.

Lemon juice, vinegar or other acids used in salad dressings and consumed with a protein meal interfere with hydrochloride secretion and, therefore, also with protein digestion.

Although nuts or cheese along with sour fruit do not constitute an ideal combination, we can accept exceptions, not only with regard to these two food items. Nuts and cheese, which contain considerable amounts of oils and fat (cream), are the only exceptions to the rule that, "when acids are eaten together with proteins, putrefaction is caused." These foods do not decompose at the same rate as other protein foods when not digested immediately. Moreover, acids do not retard the digestion of nuts and cheese as these foods contain fat in such quantities as to prevent gastric secretion longer than acids.

3.5 The combination of fat and protein

In his Physology in Modern Medecine, McLeod says: <<Fat has been shown to exert a considerable inhibitory effect on the secretion of gastric juice... **the presence of oil in the stomach delays the secretion of juice for a subsequent meal which would otherwise appear easily digested**>>. Here is an important physiological truth, the significance of which has often been overlooked. Most people who are concerned with food combinations are **unaware of the detrimental effect that fat has on gastric secretion.**

The presence of fat in the food decreases the amount of secretion that is put into the stomach, the amount of "chemical secretion" produced, the activity of the gastric glands, the amount of pepsin and hydrochloric acid in the gastric juice, and can decrease gastric tone by up to fifty percent. **This inhibitory effect may last for two or more hours.**

This means that **when protein food is ingested, fats should not be part of the menu of the same meal**. In other words, foods such as cream, butter, **various kinds of oils,** sauces, fatty meats, etc., **should not be eaten together with nuts,** cheese, eggs, or meat. It should be noted, in this regard, that foods that normally contain fat, such as nuts or cheese or milk, take longer to digest than protein foods that do not.

Our fourth rule, therefore, is "Eat fat and protein in separate meals."

It is good to know that a large amount of vegetables, especially raw, cancels out the inhibitory effects of fat, so that if you eat fats and proteins together, you can limit the damaging effects on protein digestion by consuming a large amount of vegetables.

3.6 Combinations of sugars and proteins

All sugars, those normally in commerce, syrups, sweet fruits, honey, etc.,

have an inhibiting effect on the secretion of gastric juice and on the mobility of the stomach. This fact explains the common admonition made by mothers to children that eating cookies before lunch "spoils the appetite." Sugars, along with proteins, hinder the digestion of the latter.

Sugars do not undergo digestion in the stomach. They are digested in the intestines. If eaten alone they are not retained in the stomach for long, but immediately passed into the intestines. When eaten with other foods, either proteins or starches, they are retained in the stomach for an extended period of time, waiting for the other foods to be digested first. **While waiting for the completion of the digestion of proteins and starches they ferment.**

From these simple arguments on digestion we draw another rule: *"Eat sugars and proteins in separate meals"*.

3.7 Combinations of sugars and starches

The digestion of starches generally begins in the mouth and continues, under normal conditions, in the stomach. Sugars undergo digestion neither in the mouth nor in the stomach, but in the small intestine. When consumed alone, sugars pass rapidly from the stomach to the intestine. When eaten with other foods, however, they are retained in the stomach for a certain period of time, that is, until the digestion of the latter is completed. Since under conditions of heat and moisture in the stomach they tend to ferment very rapidly, a diet of this kind will undoubtedly cause acid fermentation.

Candies, jams, jellies, commercially available sugars (white, dark, brown, etc.), honey, molasses, syrups, etc., added to cakes, bread, pastries, cereals, potatoes, etc., produce fermentation. The regularity with which millions of people eat cereal and sugar for breakfast and, as a result suffer from acidity of the stomach or other symptoms of indigestion, would be amusing if there were not some tragedy in it. **Sweet fruit with starches also causes fermentation. Those types of bread that contain dates, raisins, figs, etc., which are very popular with healthy eating advocates, are actually very harmful.** Many people claim that using honey instead of sugar can solve the problem, but this is not true. **Honey on hot desserts, syrups on hot desserts, etc., will surely ferment.**

There are many reasons for believing that the presence of sugar together with starch interferes with the digestion of the latter. When sugar is introduced into the mouth, an abundant secretion of saliva is caused, which is, however, devoid of ptyalin, as this does not act upon sugars. If starch is counterfeited with sugar, honey, jam, etc., the adaptation of the saliva to its digestion is hindered. Little, if any, will, therefore, be the quality of ptyalin secreted, and, therefore, the digestion of the starch cannot take place.

Major Reginald F. E. Austin, M.B., R.A.M.C., M.R.C.S., L.R.C.P., says: "Foods which are in themselves complete, or which become so in certain combinations, will hardly get along ideally when eaten with others . For example, bread and butter go well together, but with the addition of sugar or jam, damage will be done. This is because the sugar will be consumed first and the transformation of starch into sugar will be delayed. Mixtures between starches and sugars cause fermentation and all the trouble that comes with it>>.

Therefore, our rule will be, "Eat starches and sugars in separate meals."

3.8 Eating melons

Many people claim that they cannot eat melons. In an attempt to appear up to date, they explain that they are "allergic" to melons. I have fed melons in large quantities to hundreds of people considered to be allergic and found that the allergy was just a figment of their imagination. **Cantaloupes are such easy-to-digest foods that even the weakest digestive system is unhindered.**

But often, after consuming a melon, disorders arise, even pain of considerable intensity. Why? These foods do not undergo digestion in the stomach. What little digestion they need takes place in the intestine. If consumed properly, they are transferred to the intestines. But, if consumed with other foods which do not need for the completion of salivary or gastric digestion, a longer stay in the stomach, they too are retained. As melons, when cut and kept warm, decompose very rapidly, they cause, when eaten with other foods, the formation of gas in the stomach and many other disorders.

Let us take a person who complains of considerable pains in the abdomen, and of other disorders whenever he eats a watermelon. He is sure that he is allergic to melons, that he absolutely cannot eat them. Well: I feed this person with a great quantity of melons, without causing the formation of gas, and without causing pain or discomfort. How do I do that? **I feed only melons. I give at each meal the quantity of melons that the person wants, using them as the only food.** Immediately the person discovers that he or she is not "allergic" to melons and can eat them without experiencing any discomfort whatsoever.

Hence our rule: "Eat melons alone".

This means that **watermelons, winter melons, cantaloupes, persimmons, lattice, longs, etc., should be eaten alone.** That is, they should not be eaten as appetizers, fruits, or snacks between meals: they should constitute the meal. It is better, in fact, to base the entire meal on them. I have also tried to have melons eaten along with fresh fruit and have found no good reason why this should not be done.

3.9 Milk should be consumed alone

In nature it is the rule that puppies of all kinds take milk without adding to it any other food. In fact, in the early stages of life, young mammals consume nothing but milk. Then comes the time when puppies begin to take milk along with other foods, but always separately. Finally, there comes a time when, after being weaned, they stop consuming milk for good.

Milk is the food of the young. There is no need to continue to consume it at the end of the normal nursing period. The dairy industry and medical science have taught us that each of us, to be well, needs at least a quart of milk a day. In other words, we should never be weaned but continue the breastfeeding period forever. This is just a commercial program that does not take into account the needs of man.

Because of its protein and fat content (the cream), milk can hardly combine ideally with other foods. It combines quite well with sour fruit. The first thing that happens when it enters the stomach is its coagulation: the milk becomes curdled. The particles of curdled milk tend to cluster around those of other foods in the stomach, isolating them against the action of gastric juice. This prevents their digestion until the curdled milk particles have been digested.

Our rule for what concerns milk is: "Consume milk alone or don't consume it at all".

In the feeding of children *a fruit meal* may be given, *followed, about half an hour later, by milk*. This should not be given together with the fruit, unless it is an acid fruit. The orthodox Jew follows an excellent dietary program when he refuses to consume milk together with meat. But **even together with cereals or other starches the use of milk appears inadvisable.**

3.10 Desserts

Desserts are eaten at the end of the meal; that is, when, as a rule, the individual has already eaten more than is necessary. Here come then the sweets, cakes, puddings, ice-creams, candied fruits, etc.; foods, these, which combine very badly with almost all those which form the meal. They serve no particular purpose, and are not at all advisable.

There is only one rule that relates to *desserts: "Desert desserts."*

Dr. Tilden used to advise people that if they just couldn't do without a dessert, they should eat it with a salad and skip the next meal. Dr. Harvey W. Wiley, once affirmed that the alimentary value of sweets is out of discussion: <<you just have to find the way to digest them>>. Certainly, eaten at the end of a meal, as is the general custom, sweets cannot be well digested. And this is true for every kind of dessert. **The cold desserts, like the ice-creams, interpose a further barrier to the digestive process, the one caused by the cold.**

CHAPTER 4 - NORMAL DIGESTION

In his Textbook of Physiology, Howell states that "in the large intestine the decomposition of proteins occurs regularly and normally". He notes that <<recognizing that fermentation by bacteria is a normal occurrence in the gastro-intestinal tract, the question that arises is whether or not this process is necessary for normal digestion and nutrition>>. Following in-depth studies on the subject and on the experiments referred to it, he does not come to definitive conclusions, but deduces that <<it seems wise to adopt the point of view of conservatives and to maintain that, while the presence of bacteria does not bring positive benefits, the organism has adapted itself to neutralize their harmful action>>.

He emphasizes the fact that bacteria which cause putrefaction break down proteins into amino acids and do not limit their action to this alone: they destroy amino acids and, as the final effect of their activity, produce poisons, such as indole, scatol, phenol, phenylpropiolic and phenylacetic acids, fatty acids, carbon dioxide, hydrogen, methane, hydrogen sulphide, etc., which are not only absorbed by the feces but are also partly absorbed and subsequently eliminated through the urine. He adds that <<many of these products are excreted by the faeces, but others are partially absorbed and subsequently eliminated through the urine>>. Finally, he says: <<It has been shown that other more or less toxic substances, belonging to the group of amines, are the product of the further action of the bacteria on the amino acids present in the protein molecules>>.

It does not seem logical to infer that such a process of toxin formation is normal or necessary in digestion. Rather, it seems to me that **Howell and the other physiologists mistook an occurrence common to many as normal**. They have not asked themselves why fermentation and putrefaction occur in the digestive tract. What are the causes? Some form of poisoning, is the answer. Howell goes further, to the point of stating: <<It is well known that excessive action of bacteria leads to intestinal troubles, such as diarrhoea, or, indeed, to far more serious interference with general nutrition, by the formation of toxic products such as amines.>> However, he does not specify what he means by the expression "excessive action of bacteria."

Several times I have repeated how I consider it insane to accept every common occurrence as a normal fact. The fact that protein putrefaction occurs in almost every civilized man, is not enough to make one consider the phenomenon normal. First it is necessary to ask and answer the question, "Why is protein putrefaction such a common occurrence?" And it is useful to ask also what is its purpose.

Are putrefaction and fermentation due to overeating, inadequate protein consumption, ingestion of wrong combinations, eating under emotional or stressful conditions (fatigue, overwork, worry, fear, anxiety, pain, fever, inflammation, etc.) that delay or suspend digestion? Are they the result of damaged digestion for a different reason? Should we always take for granted the eating habits of modern man? Why should we consider as normal the findings verified in weak and sick human beings?

Feces that are unclean, slow, too hard, gas in the stomach, colitis, hemorrhoids, blood in the stool, and other facts of the same nature that accompany daily living, are held to be normal on the principle that putrefaction is a normal occurrence in the human colon. One is convinced that "whatever the reason, surely it is the right one."

The fact that there are animals whose intestinal tract is free from protein putrefaction, that there **are men whose dietary and living habits produce odorless stools and no gas in the stomach,** that a change in habits leads to a change in results, seem worthless to those physiologists who regard disorders as normal merely because they appear widespread. According to Howell the widespread septic condition of the colon in many men is normal; he completely ignores the causes which produce and maintain this state of sepsis.

The blood should receive from the digestive tract water, amino acids, fatty acids, glycerine, monosaccharides, minerals and vitamins. It should not receive alcohol, ptomains, leucomains, hydrogen sulphide, etc.: from the digestive tract, in short, nutritive materials should be received, not poisons.

When starches and complex sugars are digested, they are transformed into simple sugars called monosaccharides which, being substances that can be used by the body, represent nourishment. **When starches and sugars are fermented they are transformed into carbon dioxide, acetic acid, alcohol and water; all of** which, with the exception of water, since they are not usable are poisons. When proteins are digested, they are broken down into amino acids, which are usable substances and therefore nutrients. When, however, they putrefy, they are transformed into a great variety of ptomaines and leucomaines which are not usable substances and are therefore poisons. As it happens for all the other alimentary factors, the enzymatic digestion, prepares the foods to be utilized by the organism; the bacterial decomposition renders them unusable to the organism. The first process provides, as a final product, the nutritive elements; the second, gives as a final result the production of poisons.

What is the purpose of consuming the theoretical number of calories needed daily and then letting them ferment and putrefy in the digestive tract? Food spoiled in such a manner produces no calories.

What is the benefit of eating plenty of protein only to have it putrefy in the gastro-intestinal tract? Proteins rendered useless do not build their own amino acids. What is the benefit of eating vitamin-rich foods only to have them break down in the stomach and intestines? Foods spoiled in this manner do not supply the body with vitamins. What nutritional benefit is derived from eating foods rich in minerals and then letting them decay in the alvino duct? Foods spoiled in this way do not supply the body with the necessary minerals. Carbohydrates that ferment in the digestive tract are converted into alcohol and acetic acid, not monosaccharides. Fats, which go rancid in the stomach and intestines, do not provide the body with the fatty acids and glycerin it needs.

In order to derive sustenance from the foods consumed, it is necessary that they be digested and not go bad.

Speaking of phenol, indole and scatol, Howell emphasized the fact that phenol (carbolic acid) after being absorbed combines in part with sulphuric acid, forming an etherate sulphate or phenolsulphuric acid, and in this form is eliminated by means of the urine. <<The same is true of cresol>> he added. Indole and scatol, after being absorbed, are converted by oxidation into indossyl and scatoxyl, after which they combine with sulphuric acid, such as phenol, and are eliminated in the urine as indossyl-sulphuric acid and scatoxyl-sulphuric acid. These poisons are often found in the urine and the amount present serves to indicate the degree of putrefaction of the intestines. That the body establishes a certain tolerance to these poisons, as to other poisons introduced into the body daily, is certain, but it seems truly foolish to claim that "the body has so adapted itself to these conditions that it can neutralize" the products of bacterial activity. Certainly the disorders which arise from the accumulation of gas in the abdomen, from the **bad breath which develops from gastro-intestinal fermentation and putrefaction, from the unpleasant odor of the feces and gases emitted are as harmful as the poisons themselves. It is well known how it is possible to have a fragrant breath, how it is possible to live without swelling and gas in the stomach and without the feces having an unpleasant smell.** I believe that instead of considering normal, almost necessary, a phenomenon common to many, it would be more intelligent to consider the causes that cause it and establish whether they are normal or not. If it is possible to eliminate the unpleasant results of fermentation and putrefaction, if it is possible to remove the accumulation of oxidizing factors from the body and eliminate these bacterial products, I believe it would be wiser to do so. If experts in the field admit that "excessive bacterial activity" can cause diarrhea or even more serious damage to the body, what can we expect from prolonged bacterial activity, perhaps not always "excessive"? I think this is a pertinent question.

Anything that reduces, slows down or even suspends the digestive processes will facilitate the activity of the bacteria. Feeding in excess (i.e., feeding beyond the enzymatic capacity), feeding when fatigued, before starting work, when too cold or too hot, when feverish, when in pain, in the presence of inflammation, in the absence of hunger pangs, when worried, anxious, frightened, altered, etc.; feeding, in all these and similar circumstances, serves to favor the bacterial decomposition of the food consumed. The use of condiments, vinegar, alcohol and other substances that delay digestion favors the bacterial decomposition of the ingested substances.

If we carefully analyze the dietary habits of the majority of the modern population, we find a thousand reasons to justify the so widespread presence of fermentation and gastro-intestinal putrefaction, without having to consider these processes normal or necessary. The causes of digestive inefficiency are manifold.

One of the most common causes of digestive deficiency put into practice by the majority of people, is the wrong combinations of food. The almost universal habit of neglecting the enzymatic limitations of the body and of feeding in a hazardous manner, is largely responsible for the indigestion which, more or less constantly, affects the population. The proof of this is contained in the fact that a diet consisting of correct combinations puts an end to indigestion. This statement should not be misunderstood. Feeding with proper combinations will serve to ameliorate and not terminate indigestion, if it is due in part to other causes. If, for example, worry is one of the main factors, it will have to be eliminated in order to restore normal digestion. It must be said, however, that worry combined with wrong combinations will cause indigestion far worse than would occur with the right combinations.

Rex Beach, once a gold prospector in Alaska, talking about those who like him had worked in the gold mines, wrote: <<We ate mostly dry bread, beans and pork. The consumption of such food caused enormous problems. The worst thing in that situation was not the howling of the wolf, or the macabre laughter of the Arctic Loon, or the plaintive cry of the mating American Elk; it was the dyspeptic vomiting of the miner. Modern physiologists, ignoring the mode of eating, which in fact is the cause, would consider this "miner's vomit," his abdominal swelling and dilatation, the consequent gastro-intestinal decomposition, the foul odor of the stool, and the presence of a large amount of gas in the stomach, normal factors. If the miner had not used Alka-Seltzer or other digestives with which to relieve pain, mask and encourage further food abuse, he would have had to manually induce the gag reflexes. Constipation, alternating with diarrhea, was very common with this type of diet.

Millions of dollars are spent annually on medicines that provide temporary relief from disorders caused by the breakdown of food in the stomach and intestines. **Thousands upon thousands of people employ a wide variety of substances in an attempt to neutralise acidity, absorb gas, eliminate pain, or even defeat the headache that is a symptom of gastric irritation.** Other substances, such as pepsin for example, are also used in an attempt to facilitate digestion. Instead of considering such habits normal, Hygienists consider them extremely abnormal. The signs of good health are well-being and peace of mind, not pain and discomfort. Normal digestion need not be accompanied by symptoms of disease.

CHAPTER 5 - HOW TO COMBINE PROTEIN... FOR DINNER

And God spoke to Moses, saying, <<I have heard the murmuring of the children of Israel: go, address them in these words , "**At sunset we shall eat meat, and at sunrise we shall be filled with bread**">>. And Moses said ... <<God will give you meat in the evening and bread to your fill in the morning>>.

Thus, the murmuring of the children of Israel gave rise to a dietary habit that has faded with the passage of time but is now rediscovered in the physiological field: that of eating foods containing protein and carbohydrates in separate meals.

It is interesting to note that Tilden suggested that at least twelve hours should elapse between protein and starch meals. The biblical passage just quoted does not indicate what other foods were consumed along with the meat, but the preparations for the Passover feast speak of **lamb combined with a large quantity of green salad**. Vegetables are the substances that combine best with protein.

We have thus learned that it is best to eat foods containing protein and carbohydrates in separate meals. The digestive processes of these two kinds of food are so different that they cannot be efficiently carried out in the same digestive cavity and at the same time. This appears so different and contrary to popular custom as to require explanation.

Digestion is that physilogical process in which the body varies its activities in relation to many factors, keeping intact the character of the food. There is one remarkable fact concerning the task performed by the digestive glands, and that is that **the digestive tract can vary its fluids and enzymes in such a way that they can be adapted to the character of the food ingested**. The following statements were taken from the second edition (1961) of the Textbook of Medicai Physiology written by Arthur C. Guyton: <<... in some parts of the gastro-intestinal tract even the types of enzymes or other elements forming the secretions are modified in relation to the type of food present>>.

Perhaps Pavlov gave much importance to this ability of the digestive tract to modify fluids and enzymes to adapt them to the types of foods consumed; a certain knowledge of this phenomenon, however, already existed before his research. This fact is, today, well known to physiologists, although neither Pavlov nor anyone else has ever attempted to make a practical application of it in everyday life. In fact, physiology seems to be a "pure science", not a subject that has a practical application in the daily life of man.

Variations in the enzymes and other elements forming the digestive secretions, in the presence of different foods, represent an attempt to bring the digestive juices into conformity with the needs of the types of foods present. They include variations in the alkalinity and acidity (pH) of the secretions, in the concentration of enzymes, in the timing of secretion, etc., in adapting these secretions to the foods ingested.

Adaptation of the juices and their enzymatic content to the character of the foods ingested is possible, however, only when the foods consumed do not appear so radically different from each other as to cause a conflict between the juices required and the time of secretions. These variations in the acid-alkaline character of the secretion, in the enzyme concentration, and in the time of secretion, are of significance only when the food is conumed alone or in combination with other foods which do not interfere with the digestive processes required for that particular kind of food.

This capacity of the digestive duct to vary its secretions in such a way as to satisfy the digestive needs of every kind of food, explains how effectively it can digest a food, such as a potato, a cereal or a legume, a combination of protein and starch, provided the potato, cereal or legume is eaten alone or with other foods which do not impede the adaptation of the juices to the food. Potatoes **and meat, potatoes and cheese, potatoes and bread, being combinations between proteins and carbohydrates, cannot be digested with the same regularity** since, the juices, cannot adapt to the needs of two foods of opposite type.

It is one thing to eat one food, however complex its nature may appear; it is another to eat two foods of "opposite" species.

The digestive juices can adapt themselves excellently to one kind of food, as to cereals, for example, which are a combination of starches and proteins, but they cannot adapt themselves to two kinds of food, as, for example, bread and cheese. To better explain the truth of these statements, Dr. Tilden used to say that **nature never produced "stuffed sandwiches."** It should seem obvious that the digestive tract of man is programmed for the digestion of natural food combinations, and certainly not for that of mixtures derived from the most disparate substances put together for consumption by modern men. Natural combinations do not cause great difficulties to the digestive system. The **problems arise from the "great binges" such as those of Christmas, New Year's Eve, August bank holiday, the consumption of sweets, cocktails (even non-alcoholic ones) etc.. Such lavish banquets often end in real epidemics of "ptomaine poisoning", diphtheria, measles, etc..**

To mix the most disparate foods, a habit common among modern men, precludes the possibility that variations in the character of the secretions may render the digestion of the meal efficient. For this reason we advise the consumption of those food combinations which offer the least conflict in the digestive process; **that is to say, we recommend that you respect your own enzyme limitations.**

In their *Principles* of Biochemistry, White, Handler, Smith and Stetten state: <<The role of saliva in the digestion of starches, in the mammal, is not certain to be due to the variable duration of contact between the enzyme and the substrate. The union of the alimentary bolus with the acid gastric juice undoubtedly interrupts the action of the salivary amylase, as this enzyme is inactivated by a low pH value. Only in those individuals deficient in the secretion of gastric Hcl (hydrochloric acid) can salivary digestion continue in the stomach˜.

The matter reported here, that the hydrochloric acid of the gastric juice prevents or even destroys salivary amylase or ptyalin in the stomach, is well known to physiologists and physiological chemists; but these, instead of frankly admitting, as the above-mentioned authors do, that **salivary digestion ends immediately when the food reaches the stomach**, tend to ignore the fact. Arthur K. Anderson, in his *The Essential Factors* of Physiological *Chemistry* (Essentials Of Physiological Chemistry; 1961), after having duly acknowledged this thesis, attempts to evade its implications, stating that: <<Because salivary amylase acts until the

pH reaches 4.0, it appears evident that significant action can take place in the stomach before sufficient acidity develops to inhibit it ... It has been proved that amylase activity can continue for thirty minutes after the ingestion of food ... >>.

Repetitions of Anderson's tests, carried out in the laboratory using a standard pH value, showed that at a pH of 4 there was no amylase activity and that there was slight amylase activity at a pH of 5. From this I deduced that amylase activity is inhibited in the stomach much earlier than Anderson claims. Research has shown that the addition of hydrochloric acid to food stops the action of ptyalin in sixty seconds. The acidity of the juice in the stomach is a factor to be taken into account, not only when the acidic juice gradually enters the food bolus, but from the moment the first mouthful of food is swallowed.

In the 1961 edition of *The* Physiological Basis of Medical Practice, physiologists Best and Taylor, state: << Salivary amylase, for its activity, requires an alkaline, neutral, or slightly acid environment; it was therefore thought that stronger acidic gastric juice would prevent or arrest salivary digestion. However, it has been shown that the final part of the meal, usually consisting of carbohydrates, can remain at the bottom of the stomach, protected against the action of the gastric juice of the layer of food previously ingested... This is the reason why it is thought that under favourable circumstances, during this period of time, good digestion of starches could be obtained... >>.

The unconscious error made by these physiologists is obvious at first glance. The carbohydrate, more or less regularly consumed at the end of the meal, is the dessert which is a sugar and, as such, does not require salivary digestion. People, as a general habit, do not eat proteins at the beginning of the meal and starches at the end: they eat them together. Just think, in this regard, of the famous sandwich with the hamburger inside. Meat and bread, bread and eggs, meat and potatoes or meat and peas are very frequent combinations.

If the physiologist appears satisfied when he obtains a "good digestion of the starches" in the upper part of the stomach, while the starches in the rest of the stomach are not digested at all, he may also consider himself satisfied in the presence of the irregular digestion which takes place following the consumption of the most popular combinations; an intelligent person, however, should not even consider such combinations. The statement made by Anderson that "every starch, not hydrolyzed in the mouth and stomach by salivary amylase, is digested in the intestine by pancreatic amylase," is contradicted by the **large quantity of undigested starch found in the faeces of those who mix proteins and carbohydrates together.**

Highly acidic gastric juices are secreted for the digestion of proteinous foods, but, if the starch is consumed without the protein, the gastric juice may appear alkaline, neutral, or slightly acid. Even if the starch contains protein, as in the case of potatoes, cereals or legumes, the acid secretion is regulated in time so that it is put into the food after the completion of salivary digestion of the starch. If we were to consume protein and starch meals at separate times, we would improve our digestion and consequently our health. Since all physiologists agree that the character of the digestive juice produced corresponds to the character of the food to be digested, it is inferred that complicated food mixtures greatly impair the efficiency of digestion. Simple meals are more easily digested, therefore they are the healthiest.

Conventional eating habits violate all the rules on food combinations which have been given in the preceding chapters, and, as it seems that most people take almost no pleasure in the frequent ailments and pains they experience, there are few who do not underestimate the importance of such habits. These persons, when the subject falls upon food combinations, generally declare that they can eat the most abstruse combinations without accusing the slightest disorder. Life and death, health and sickness are for them purely accidental circumstances. Unfortunately, their point of view is also encouraged by medical science.

More than sixty years of feeding the healthy and the sick, the weak and the strong, the old and the young, have shown that any change in dietary habits is immediately followed by an improvement in health, as a result of the lightening of the work done by the digestive organs. Thus, with the improvement of digestion and nutrition, toxic factors also disappear. I can further say, from experience, that such meals are followed by less fermentation and putrefaction, less air in the stomach, and fewer disturbances. I do not believe that experiences are of much value if they cannot be explained in principles, but, for my part, this has been done in the preceding pages; my experiences, therefore, assume considerable value. The rules on food combinations presented here are rooted in physiology, have been proved by experience, and may, therefore, be considered of value.

Much of the **annual massacre of the tonsils of children** arises from a state of constant fermentation in the digestive tract as a result of their constant feeding of meat and bread, cereals and sugar, cookies and fruit, etc. Until parents learn to feed their children while respecting their enzyme limitations, they will continue to suffer not only from colds and tonsils, but also from gastritis (indigestion), diarrhea, constipation, fever, various "childhood diseases," polio, etc., etc,

The most common combinations are bread and meat (hamburger buns, sausage buns, etc.), bread and eggs, bread and cheese, potatoes and meat, potatoes and eggs (eggs in potato salad, for example), cereal and eggs (at breakfast), etc. **There is no habit of eating foods containing protein first and then carbohydrates.** They are consumed together and thrown into the stomach in the most haphazard and incorrect manner. The common way of preparing breakfast is to eat cereal first (with milk, cream, or sugar), then eggs with bread. Bearing in mind the manner in which the majority of Americans prepare their breakfast, one should not be surprised at the large number of cases of indigestion which occur, and at the extensive consumption of Alka-Seltzer, Diger-Seltz, and other kinds of digestives.

Italian dishes that are rapidly spreading in America generally consist of spaghetti with meatballs, spaghetti and cheese, or ravioli. Spaghetti is usually served with tomato sauce and bread. The salad cut into small pieces, which serves as a side dish, is dressed with plenty of olive oil, vinegar and salt. It often also contains other types of condiments. Bread usually accompanies it. Margarine is also often served to spread on bread. Beer or wine are the traditional drinks for such a meal.

The radio announcer advises those who are victims of their bad eating habits, in cases of "acid indigestion," to have recourse to one of the many digestive aids on the market; no one ever dreams of saying that such palliative means guarantee the progression of bad habits causing, later on, the recurrence of the disorders even in a more serious manner.

"From the small acorn comes the big oak," says an old maxim, but in pathology this principle is never applied.

Since, physiologically speaking, the first step in the digestion of starches and proteins takes place in opposite environments - the former need an alkaline environment and the latter an acid environment - foods containing these two types of substances should never be ingested at the same time.

Physicists know that **undigested starches absorb pepsin**. Considering this fact, one inevitably deduces that eating starches and proteins during the same meal will serve to delay the digestion of the latter. Some say, on the basis of supposed experiments, that this delay is not so great, as the digestion of proteins takes place only after four or six minutes; an insignificant time, therefore. There is reason to believe, however, that these assertions are erroneous; for if the only results of those combinations were the four or six minutes' delay found in the digestion of the proteins, there should not be found in the faeces of those who had consumed those mixtures a large quantity of undigested proteins. I am convinced, therefore, that the interference with the digestion of proteins is far greater than that indicated by the experiments. Those who do not understand the efforts to propagate healthier habits of eating tend to concentrate their attention on proteins, and, using the results of these experiments as a basis on which to build their objections to the union of proteins and carbohydrates, avoid considering the interruption resulting from such mixtures in the digestion of starches.

We have previously learned that it is unwise to consume foods containing more than one type of protein, both because this complicates and delays the digestive process and because it would lead to an excess of protein. At **present there is a tendency to exaggerate the need for protein and to encourage its excessive consumption**. I would like to discourage this and point out that such behaviour would only repeat what was seen hundreds of years ago. Indeed, dietary fads seem to repeat themselves periodically.

The specific secretions relating to each kind of food are so different in character that Pavlov spoke of a "juice of milk," a "juice of bread," and a "juice of meat." Two proteins of different character and composition require different kinds of digestive juices, and these juices, of different intensity and character, are introduced into the stomach at different times or during the digestive process.

Khizhin, one of Pavlov's collaborators, showed that the secretory response of the glands is "not limited to the characteristics of the juice, but extends to the rate of flow and also to its total quantity." The character of the food consumed determines not only the digestive capacity of the juice secreted on it, but also its total acidity: acidity, which is higher with meat and lower with bread. There is also an extraordinary adaptation of the juice in regard to its timing: the strongest juice is secreted during the first hour for meat, during the third for bread, and during the last hour of digestion for milk.

Owing to the circumstance that each separate kind of food determines a definite hourly rate of secretion, and causes limitations in the various capacities of the juices, those foods which require considerable differences in digestive secretions, as, for instance, bread and meat, should by no means be consumed at the same meal. Pavlov showed that five times as much pepsin is secreted on bread as on milk, and this, however, contains a quantity of protein equivalent to that of bread; the nitrogen, on the other hand, present in meat requires more pepsin than milk. These different kinds of food received quantities of enzymes corresponding to the differences in their digestibility. Comparing two quantities of equal weight, meat requires the most gastric juice and milk the least, but comparing the same quantities of nitrogen, bread requires more juice and meat less.

Physiologists are aware of these phenomena, but have never attempted to apply them in any way. Indeed, when they do consent to discuss them in connection with the practical problems of (food) life, they tend to take the subject at arms length and to give flimsy reasons which are supposed to be intended to keep up the bad habits which, almost everywhere, seem to be in fashion. They appear inclined to regard as normal, as we have hinted in the preceding chapter, the immediate harm which results from such harmful dietary practices.

Because of the inhibitory effects on the digestive secretion of acids, sugars and fats, it is not advisable to consume foods containing these substances together with proteins. Let us briefly consider these combinations.

The inhibitory effect of fat (butter, cream, oils, margarine, etc.) on gastric secretion, delaying the digestion of proteins for two hours or more, makes us realize that fats should not be consumed along with proteins. The presence of fat in fried meat, fried eggs, milk, nuts, and foods similar to these, is the probable reason why these foods require a longer digestive period than that required by a lean roast, boiled lean meat, or poached eggs. **Fatty meat and fried meat cause not inconsiderable harm to those who use them. It should, therefore, be a rule not to eat fats together with proteins.**

The inhibiting effect of fat on gastric secretion can be counterbalanced by consuming a large quantity of fresh, and especially raw, vegetables. Raw cabbage is particularly effective in this case. For this reason it would be better to consume vegetables together with cheese or nuts rather than together with sour fruit, although this is not particularly discouraged.

Sugars, by inhibiting both gastric secretion and mobility (the movement of the stomach), interfere with the digestion of proteins. At the same time, these substances, which do not require digestion in the mouth and stomach, remain pending the completion of protein digestion and therefore ferment. Proteins should never be consumed together with sugars. Experiments conducted by Dr. Phillip Norman showed that the consumption of cream and sugar at the end of a meal delayed digestion for several hours.

Acids, of any kind, inhibit the secretion of gastric juice. Therefore they also interfere in the digestion of proteins. The **exceptions are cheese, nuts and avocados**. These foods, contending cream and oil inhibit the secretion of gastric juices in the same way as acids, are not disturbed in digestion when eaten together with acids.

The **foods that combine best with those containing protein are non-starchy, juicy vegetables**: spinach, thistles, kale, green beets, green turnips, Chinese cabbage, broccoli, asparagus, fresh green beans, okra, Brussels sprouts, squash, onions, celery, lettuce, cucumber, radishes, watercress, parsley, endive, dandelion, collard greens, turnip greens, escarole, carduccia, broccoli rabe, bamboo shoots and other similar non-starchy foods.

The following vegetables, on the other hand, combine very poorly with protein: beets, turnips, pumpkins, carrots, sassefriga (scorzonera root and fruit), cauliflower, kohlrabi, turnip, beans, peas, artichokes, potatoes (including sweet potatoes). These foods, containing starch, combine best with foods containing starchy substances. Beans and peas, being in themselves combinations of proteins and starches should be used either as starches or as proteins and

combined with fresh vegetables, without the addition of other starches or other proteins. Potatoes are sufficiently starchy to be eaten alone.

The following menus [1] are ideally combined protein meals. It is recommended that the protein meal be eaten in the evening. **Acids, oils and condiments should not be consumed with the protein meal.** Quantities are left to the individual's choice.

$$\left\{\begin{array}{l}\text{Insalata}\\ \text{Zucca verde}\\ \text{Spinaci}\\ \text{Noci}\end{array}\right.\quad\text{... è il primo esempio di menù, seguono gli altri ...}$$

Salad, Green cabbage, Yellow pumpkin, Avocado,
Salad, Spinach, Green pumpkin, Cheese flakes,
Salad, Thistles, Asparagus, Walnuts,
Salad, Mustard sprouts, Fresh beans, Avocado,
Salad, Beet sprouts, Fresh peas, Cheese flakes
Salad, Beets, Broccoli, Walnuts, Avocado, Cheese flakes
Salad, Broccoli, Fresh corn, Walnuts,
Salad, Yellow pumpkin, Cabbage, Sunflower seeds ,
Salad, Spinach, Cabbage, Whole cheese
Salad, Abelmosco, Spinach, Walnuts,
Salad, Spinach, Broccoli, Sunflower seeds,
Salad , Baked aubergines , Thistles , Eggs
Salad, Thistles, Yellow pumpkin, Walnuts,
Salad, Thistles, Abelmosco, Cheese flakes,
Salad, Spinach, Yellow pumpkin, Eggs
Salad, Beets, Green beans, Walnuts,
Salad, Abelmosco, Yellow pumpkin, Cheese flakes,
Salad, Turnips, Green beans, Eggs
Salad, Thistles, Yellow pumpkin, Lamb chops,

Salad, Thistles, Yellow pumpkin, Avocado,
Salad, Abelmosco, Red cabbage, Avocado
Salad, Green pumpkin, Green cabbage, Whole cheese,
Salad, Cabbage, Spinach, Walnuts,
Salad, Asparagus, Artichokes, Avocado
Salad, Beets, Abelmosco, Sunflower seeds,
Salad, Broccoli, Fresh beans, Walnuts,
Salad, Yellow pumpkin, Thistles, Avocado,
Salad, Green cabbage, Green beans, Sunflower seeds,
Salad, Steamed onions, Thistles, Whole cheese,
Salad, Baked aubergines, Green cabbage, Avocado
Salad, Baked aubergines ,Thistles, Soybean sprouts ,
Salad, Green pumpkin, Turnips, Roast beef,
Salad, Yellow pumpkin, Mustard sprouts, American walnuts
Salad, Asparagus, Fresh beans, Walnuts,
Salad, Red cabbage, Spinach, Cheese flakes,
Salad, Green beans, Abelmosco, Barbecued lamb
Salad, Abelmosco, Beets, Sunflower seeds,
Salad, Asparagus, Broccoli, Eggs,
Salad, Brussels sprouts, Green cabbage, Walnuts

1always starts with salad, 4 foods per menu. This is dinner!

CHAPTER 6 - HOW TO COMBINE STARCHES... FOR LUNCH

There are those who say, <<Do not serve more than two foods high in sugar or starch during the same meal. If you serve bread and potatoes together, the allowable limit of starches far exceeds the normal level. A meal that includes peas, bread, potatoes, sugar, dessert, and finally, mint, should also include vitamin B complex capsules, baking soda (different from that used on vegetables), and the address of the nearest specialist in arthritis or other degenerative diseases>>.

For more than seventy years it has been a rule of Hygienist circles to eat **only one starchy food per meal and not to add to it any other food containing sugar. Sugars, syrups, honey, cakes, chocolate, have been banned from meals containing starchy substances.** To those who ask us for advice, we do not say to eat sugars together with starches and then take soda. We advise avoiding fermentation which is almost inevitable under those circumstances. In hygienic circles it is considered an **act of foolishness to ingest a poison and then use an antidote to try to nullify its effects.** Therefore, in our opinion, the best thing is to avoid the consumption of the poison.

Sugars with starches cause **fermentation. This is synonymous with stomach acidity** which, in turn, means discomfort. Those who habitually consume honey considering it a "natural sweetener" should know that the rule of not consuming sugars and starches together also refers to honey. **Honey or syrup, it makes no difference, together with cereals they cause fermentation.** White sugar, dark sugar, "raw" sugar, dark sugar imitations (i.e. colored white sugar), black molasses or other types of sweetening syrups, combined with starches cause fermentation. Soda can neutralize the resulting acid, but it cannot stop fermentation.

For over sixty years it has been the custom of members of Hygienist circles to **consume a large quantity of green salad (without tomatoes or other acid substances) along with starches.** The salad should be eaten in large quantities and should consist of fresh, raw vegetables. Such a composed type of salad contains a plethora of vitamins and minerals. The vitamins contained in these vegetables are genuine products and not imitations created in a laboratory. No "equally good and valid" imitation has ever been able to satisfy the Hygienist. **For us there is only the natural product, we do not accept any reproduction.** Capsule feeding is just a commercial program launched by the drug industry.

Vitamins complement each other. Man needs not only vitamin B complex, but all existing ones. A large amount of green salad in its natural state, for example, provides several types of vitamins, including those not yet discovered by man. Vitamins not only cooperate with each other in the nutritional process, but also with minerals in the body. These are provided by vegetables. Ingesting prepared vitamins, along with calcium or iron, will not achieve the same purpose. Minerals thus presented, are not usable. There is, in fact, no better source of food substances than the vegetable kingdom; for chemical laboratories have not hitherto been able to supply food as nutritious. Hygienists recommend only one starch per meal, not because there is any conflict as to the digestion of these substances, but because to **use two or more starches in the same meal would lead to an excessive consumption of such food**. It is better, especially in the diet of the sick, to limit the consumption of starches to one per day. Persons endowed with extraordinary powers of self-control may be able to afford the consumption of food containing two starches, but such individuals are very rare, so the rule should be: *'only one starch per meal'*.

The same author says: <<Whether you're eating a hamburger from the sleaziest place or a fillet steak from the most luxurious restaurant, you're always consuming protein. Whether it's a pancake from a cheap café or a crépe suzette from a fancy place, you're always eating carbohydrates. And whether it's margarine or butter, you are always consuming fat. These are the three basic substances in foods; the fourth is the bran. Every food is made up of a majority of one of these three substances. Some highly refined foods, such as sugar, contain only one of these three substances, but, generally speaking, foods contain all of them>>.

We, however, do not hold it to be true that the fourth part of a food is the bran, as this is not a food; nor is it true that all foods show a preponderance in any one of these four substances. **Young growing plants, in fact, do not contain much bran, as their cellulose is nearly all digestible.** They are especially important for minerals and vitamins. Excluded from its "big four" are the minerals which are found abundantly in almost all foods. Reading the preceding quotation, one might easily infer that one protein may be considered as good as another, one fat as good as another, and that any combination of foods, such as hamburger or tenderloin, is as good as any other; one might conclude, therefore, that foods may be prepared in the manner one pleases. The author has not expressed these notions; yet his statements might easily lead the reader to believe that any kind of diet is valid.

What I want to point out is that, generally, almost all foods contain carbohydrates, fats, proteins, and bran, and that this makes the prohibition on combinations of starches and proteins valid. **Of course, there is a big difference between natural combinations and the artificial ones routinely consumed. The digestive tract of man is such that it can digest natural combinations, but it is certainly not adapted to digest those complicated combinations much in use among modern populations.** The natural combinations do not cause great problems to the digestive system, but, one thing is to eat only one food even if of a complex nature, and another is to eat two of "opposite species". The digestive juices are immediately adapted to a single food, such as cereals, which are a combination of starches and proteins; they cannot, however, be adapted to two foods, such as bread and cheese. Tilden, in fact, very often reminded people that nature does not produce stuffed sandwiches.

It should become apparent that our digestive system is only adapted for the digestion of natural combinations and that for the others, the artificial ones, it presents difficulties. The eating habits of modern people are so far from resembling natural products that it is impossible to regard them as normal.

The author quoted above seemed to ignore the problem of food combinations only because he had not carefully studied the digestive process. It is true that nature provides certain combinations. It is true that such combinations cause little difficulty to digestion. But, and this is the point which escapes almost all dieticians, the organism is capable of adapting the digestive secretions, as regards capacity and acidity, concentration of enzymes and time of secretion, only to the digestive requirements of one particular food, and such adaptation of the juices is not possible in the presence of two different kinds of food. The physiologist Cannon showed that if starch is mixed with saliva, its digestion continues in the stomach for at least two hours. Of course, this does not happen when, together with acids, proteins are ingested, for in this case, the glands of the stomach produce much acid gastric juice with which they flood the food, thus interrupting salivary gastric digestion.

He states that the purpose of saliva is to initiate the digestive process of starches. "That is why," he adds, "one should chew bread, cereals, and other starchy foods very thoroughly; that is why one should not drink water while eating. For, although water, during meals, is not altogether contraindicated in that it helps the body in the process of digestion, it must not be allowed to weaken, in the mouth, the action of the saliva on the starches>>.

The digestion of starches begins, or should begin, in the mouth; however, they are retained here for such a short time that digestion is not possible. **If the starches are consumed in the proper manner, their salivary digestion will continue in the stomach.** If acids or proteins are ingested with them, their digestion will be inhibited if not entirely suspended. Drinking water during the meal will result in the weakening of the action of the saliva on the starches in the stomach and mouth, and in any case, water, is not obligatory to facilitate the digestion of food. It **is better to drink it ten or fifteen minutes before the meal**, because, if it is done while eating, it dilutes the digestive juices and, passing through the stomach, takes them and the enzymes with it.

The following menus represent properly combined starchy meals. It is suggested that they be consumed at lunchtime. Starches should be eaten dry and be chewed and inhaled before swallowing. No acids should be consumed with a starch meal. Our advice, therefore, is to eat a large protein-based salad in the evening and a smaller starch-based salad at lunch. The individual may eat as much as he wishes.

$$\begin{cases} \text{Insalata} \\ \text{Rape} \\ \text{Zucca gialla} \\ \text{Castagne} \end{cases} \ldots \text{è il primo esempio di menù, seguono gli altri} \ldots$$

Salad, Spinach, Red cabbage, Roots of Caladium,
Salad, Beets, Gombo, Baked dark rice,
Salad, Spinach, Green beans, Coconut,
Salad, Green beans, Baked aubergines, Boiled Caladium roots,
Salad, Turnips, Asparagus, Dark rice,
Salad, Green beans Navon cabbage, Potatoes,
Salad, Turnips, Gombo, Artichokes,
Salad, Green cabbage, Fresh corn, Dark rice,
Salad, Spinach, Beets, Potatoes,
Salad, Savoy cabbage, Gombo, Artichokes,
Salad, Beets, Cauliflower, Baked pumpkin
Salad, Green beans, Turnips, Sweet potatoes,
Salad, Spinach, Turnips, Artichokes,
Salad, Beans, Gombo, Baked pumpkin,
Salad, Asparagus, White pumpkin, Yam (Puerto Rican potatoes),
Salad, Gombo, Green beans, Artichokes,
Salad, Turnips, Broccoli, American peanuts
Salad, Beets, Cauliflower, Sweet potatoes,
Salad, Spinach, Cabbage, Chestnuts,
Salad, Peas, Carrots, Parsnips
Salad, Asparagus, Gombo, American peanuts,
Salad, Thistles, Peas, Pumpkin,
Salad, Thistles, Green beans, American peanuts
Salad, Gombo, Beets, Wholemeal bread,
Salad, Green beans, Broccoli, Pumpkin,
Salad, Spinach, Green beans, Dark rice
Salad, Yellow beans, Savoy cabbage, Potatoes,
Salad, Spinach, Cabbage, Baked pumpkin,
Salad, Thistles, Gombo, Dark rice
Salad, Green beans, Yellow pumpkin ,Potatoes,
Salad, Beets, Yellow pumpkin, Potatoes,
Salad, Thistles, Asparagus, Baked beans
Salad, Gombo, Brussels sprouts, Potatoes,
Salad, Savoy cabbage, Gombo, Dark rice,

Salad, Thistles, Yellow pumpkin, Oven-baked Caladium roots
Salad, Green beans, Cabbage, Sweet potatoes,
Salad, Spinach, Beans, American peanuts,
Salad, Gombo, Beets, Boiled caladium roots 1

CHAPTER 7 - HOW TO EAT FRUIT... FOR BREAKFAST

William Henry Porter, M.D., in his book Eating to Live Longer, states that the consumption of fruit <<is one of the most dangerous dietary follies>>, but admits that eaten alone it does no harm. I am sure that if he were called upon to discuss food combinations he would consider the subject a waste of time. Dr. Percy Howe of Harvard noted that people who were troubled by eating oranges at the end of meals were perfectly well if they ate the fruit alone. Dr. Dewey, an expert in fasting, was against the consumption of the fruit because, he declared, it impaired digestion. None of these people knew the combination of foods. They **simply noticed that fruit, together with other foods, caused damage;** however, they did not blame the other foods for this, but the fruit. There is no reason, however, to consider fruit more harmful than all those foods that are eaten together with it.

Man, the archetypal "cheiroteira," should develop those frugivorous habits peculiar to his anatomical structure, and from which, during the course of years, he has considerably detached himself, perhaps owing to his wandering after the abandonment of his endogenous home in the warmer regions. His sense of taste, the expression of an organic demand, must, of course, be present in health as well as in sickness; **the taste which now demands meat, will give way to a more exquisite appreciation of the delicate flavours of fruits, vegetables, and the different kinds of nuts and hazelnuts in all possible combinations, satisfying both the eye and the nose and mouth.**

Fruit can be considered one of the best foods. Nothing is more pleasant than eating a good apple, a ripe banana, a creamy avocado or sweet, ripe grapes. A peach that has reached the right point of ripeness brings real pleasure to the palate. Fruit is a real treasure trove of eating pleasure. With its range of delicate flavours, delicious aromas and colours that are pleasing to the eye, it is always an invitation to eating pleasure.

Fruit is not only a joy to the eye, nose or mouth: it is a perfect mixture of pure and nutritious elements. Only some types of fruit are rich in protein, such as avocados and olives, but all are full of sugars; others contain acids, minerals and vitamins. **Together with nuts (which, botanically, are classified as fruit) and vegetables, fruit constitutes an adequate diet: in fact, these foods constitute the ideal diet** for the normally fruitarian animal that is man. Eating fruit is a great pleasure. Mother Nature has flavoured it in such a way as to make its consumption very pleasant. There are a thousand reasons for urging us to eat these foods which Mother Nature has so richly filled with pleasant tastes and intact nutrients.

Nothing is more pleasant than **a meal of fruit. Such a** meal is always an invitation to pleasure, and never causes the problems which may arise when such foods are eaten with others. It also does not harm the digestion, is good for you, and is refreshing and nourishing. The exquisite joy of eating such a natural meal, the wonderful feeling of well-being that follows, the genuine sense of satisfaction, far surpasses the sensations experienced when eating other foods.

This is, therefore, the ideal way to eat fruit: eat it as a meal, and on its own The acids and sugars contained in fruit do not combine well with starches and proteins; the oils in avocados or olives do not combine well with proteins. Why, then, risk digestive problems by eating fruit along with meat, eggs, bread, etc.?

Fruit undergoes almost no digestion in the mouth and stomach, and, as a rule, is rapidly introduced into the intestine where the minimum digestive process necessary to it takes place. To eat it together with other foods which require, in the stomach, longer times of digestion, is to retain it unnecessarily until the digestion of other foods is completed. This causes bacterial decomposition. Previously we have already talked about this phenomenon in relation to the melons, which are also fruits.

One should not eat fruit in the intervals between meals. To do so is to put stuff into the stomach when it is still engaged in digesting the previous meal. Disorders are sure to arise. Our rule, therefore, from which we should not deviate, is to *"eat meals of fruit without accompanying them with other foods."*

The habit of drinking a large quantity of fruit juice between meals (lemon, orange, grapefruit, grape, tomato, papaya, etc.), is the cause of the many indigestions manifested by those who are convinced that they are feeding themselves in the right way. This habit, now rediscovered, was quite in vogue in hygienic circles some sixty or eighty years ago, and the effects it caused compelled many people to abandon the innovative diet and return to meat diets. I want to quote Dr. Robert Walter's experience with fruit juices, mentioned in his Exact Science of *Health*. He states that as a result of the treatments he had undergone in an attempt to restore himself (first medical and then hydropathic) he developed first an "insatiable appetite for food" and later, after an irritation in the stomach, "a gluttony which no amount of food could satisfy". He added, "my thirst was considerable, but I did not want water, and since I had always been told about the superior quality of fruit, I continually asked to drink refreshing juices. These, however, fermented in my stomach, creating and perpetuating the troubles which they only temporarily succeeded in relieving, keeping me in a state of constant fever and hunger which no other kind of suffering has ever equalled."

As a result, the doctor abandoned his vegetarian practices and returned to eating meat. Because he ate at all hours of the day (drinking fruit juice means eating) he had developed a neurosis which he mistakenly mistook for hunger. Trying to satisfy a neurosis by eating is like trying to put out a fire with gasoline. **Those who confuse gastric irritation with hunger pangs and try to satisfy it by using the very causes of the irritation will see their situation quickly worsen.** Abandoning vegetarian practices saved Dr. Walter, not because vegetarianism is wrong, but because he began to eat only one meal a day and ceased "stuffing" himself with fruit juices at meals.

No diet can be beneficial if it is ruined by the consumption of fruit juices. This is not because fruit juices are bad in themselves - they are in fact very good - but because, if used excessively, they damage the digestion. Many of the mistakes made by the so-called dieticians could be avoided by a glance at the history of dietetic reform. All their "discoveries" were implemented and applied long ago, and several of the most popular ones today had already been tried and abandoned as harmful.

Although green vegetables form the ideal combination with nuts, sour fruits are not altogether inadvisable with these foods; we say, therefore, that they may be eaten together with them.

Of course this pertains to protein nuts, not starchy ones like coconut, chestnuts, acorns, etc. Sweet fruits and nuts, despite the delicious flavor they produce, form a combination that needs to be questioned.

Avocados, which contain more protein than milk, should not be combined with other proteins. Rich in fat, they also inhibit the digestion of other proteins. **There is no objection to combining them with acidic fruits. They should not, however, be consumed with either sweet fruits or nuts.** Many maintain that papaya aids the digestion of proteins, and for this reason should be consumed with them. Such a combination is not correct, and even if it is true, as is claimed, that papaya contains an enzyme which digests proteins, this is a further reason for not combining it with other proteins. **The use of "digestives," inevitably weakens the digestive capacity of the individual.** If the digestion is found to be damaged, the cause(s) of the damage must be removed and then provide the digestive system with the necessary rest to become regular again.

The following menus are proper fruit combinations and are **recommended to be eaten in the morning . Do not add sugar to fruit.** All varieties of fruit in season can be used. The quantity is left to the individual's choice.

$$\begin{cases} \text{Arance} \\ \text{Pompelmo} \end{cases} \ldots \text{ è il primo menù, seguono gli altri} \ldots$$

Fresh figs, Peaches,
Apricots, Mango,
Cherries, Apricots,
Oranges, Pineapple,
Cherries, Apricots,
Plums, Cherries,
Peaches, Nectarines,
Grapefruit, Apples,
Bananas, Pears,
Grapes, Oranges with cream,

Mango, Cherries,
Apricots, Bananas,
Khaki, Dates,
Apples, Grapes,
Dates, A glass of sour milk,
Papaya, Khaki,
Dates, Apples,
Pears, Bananas,
Pears, Figs,
A glass of sour milk, Apples,
Grapes, Figs,

As a variation to these menus, you can prepare a tasty protein fruit salad in the following way:

A **fruit salad** consisting of: Grapefruit, Orange, Apple, Pineapple, Lettuce, Celery, Four ounces of cottage cheese or four ounces of walnuts, or a larger amount of avocado.

In spring, the fruit salad can be composed of seasonal fruit: Peaches, Plums, Apricots, Cherries, Nectarines, **Lettuce, Celery**.

Sweet fruits - bananas, raisins, dates, figs, prunes, etc. - should not be consumed in fruit salad if you want to ingest protein.

CHAPTER 8 - A SALAD A DAY

A good quantity of salad at every meal is one of the most important elements of the diet. In the prevention of disease it is far superior to all the vaccines and serums hitherto employed. The consumption of salads, at least in this country, is a recent innovation which has its origins among those who are constantly in search of new kinds of diets. **The addition of a properly prepared salad to a meal improves its nutritional value.**

At the beginning of the century the eating habits were certainly worse than they appear today: meat, bread and potatoes were eaten three times a day with the addition of sweets, desserts, etc., in combinations and in abominable quantities that could constitute the right meal for a boar of three hundred kilos. These were times when meat, bread, and potatoes, together with many other side foods such as butter, cream, mayonnaise, sugar, and sweets in general, were the most common tastes of the people. Fresh fruit and vegetables had little place in the diets of most people. In those days, "medical" science was shocked at the thought of eating raw vegetables or fresh fruit. They contained germs! <<All raw vegetables contain typhoid germs>>, they said. But, in the footsteps of the "eccentrics" and "healers", people learned to eat food in its natural state, abandoning the fear of germs. Eating such foods, however, no cases of typhoid occurred. Today, even the most bacteriophobic doctors eat raw vegetables. The only food that everyone refuses to consume without prior sterilization (because it contains typhoid and tubercular germs) is milk.

Although the way of eating has improved compared to the past, people still tend to overdo what they consume. It has reduced to some extent the work of the stomach and intestines but at the expense of the liver, pancreas, and endocrine glands. Today, people consume large quantities of raw fruits and vegetables. Lettuce, cucumbers, celery, apples, strawberries, citrus fruits, etc., are grown in huge quantities and transported all over the country. Trains laden with lettuce have now been substituted for the wheelbarrows that were once used to transport it.

I remember that until not too long ago, "doctors" categorically discouraged the use of "natural" vegetables and fruits because of the germs they contained. Until it was discovered that fresh vegetables and fruits were the best sources of vitamins (and this discovery was only reached after doctors themselves were forced to admit that people on raw vegetable and fruit diets improved dramatically), they continued to warn people about the dangers of eating these foods. Indeed, in some countries such as Mexico, India and China, such preconceptions still exist. Nature provides her products in a state of physiological equilibrium; therefore, when they are used without having undergone any kind of alteration, one is sure that no harm is done to the organism. But, when portions are extracted from such products, when sugar is extracted from cane or beet, and flour from wheat, one comes into contact with artificial products to which the natural equilibrium has been lost, and which are devoid of the essential elements of nutrition. The remedy for such a situation is to **eat the natural, raw foods produced from fertile soil.**

A salad of raw, non-starchy vegetables should accompany every protein and starchy meal. The habit of eating shrimp, potato or other similar salads does not achieve the goal. In fact, such dishes do not even deserve the name of salads. Salads should consist of lettuce, celery, cucumbers, green and red peppers (the non-starchy varieties), cabbage, tomatoes, and other non-starchy vegetables. Foods should be fresh and not seasoned with salt, vinegar, oil, mayonnaise, or substances of that nature. Tomatoes should be included in salads only when protein, not starches, is being consumed in the meal. Bitter foods such as onions, garlic, watercress, radishes and others are not recommended either as ingredients in a salad or on their own.

To ensure a complete intake of minerals and vitamins, a salad of the above type should be eaten with each protein or carbohydrate meal. The salad usually served in restaurants consists of two leaves of lettuce, a slice of half-ripe tomato, and the whole covered with a radish, a spicy olive and a good dose of dressing; such a combination is not only not correct but would not even satisfy the vitamin and mineral needs of a canary. **The salad should be the most agreeable part of the meal**, and it can only be so if the choice of its materials is appropriate.

I created this saying, "a salad a day keeps acidosis away". This is true, however, only for those salads combined properly. Shrimp salads, potato salads, egg salads, and salads covered in oil and vinegar cannot be considered as such.

The term "salad" comes from a Latin word meaning salt, and our vegetables contain an abundance of minerals in the most directly assimilable form. In a diet there are no substitute foods for vegetables. It is important that the majority of them be eaten, if at all, in their natural state (raw). In **general, the green leaves of plants are the richest sources of organic salts (minerals) and vitamins; they contain small amounts of the highest-grade proteins and are the best sources of chlorophyll, which, although it does** not serve to deodorize the breath or the body, **is essential in the nutrition of animals.**

Salads do not appear to be of extreme importance in the diets of those who eat mainly raw foods and large amounts of fruits and vegetables. Those who eat a lot of meat, grains, legumes and other starchy, high-protein foods should eat one to two plates of salad daily.

An English author affirms: <<two or three hundred years ago, our ancestors, devourers of meat, could 'dust off' a fifteen-course meal without the slightest shadow of fruit; from duck to chicken, from pig to pheasant, from fish to meat again, to the point, sometimes, of even dying of indigestion or apoplexy. Some tribes of Native American Indians, who fed almost exclusively on meat, considered fruit and vegetables to be women's food, while, some hunters of Asia or Africa, though very few in number, made no use of them at all>>. Eating a salad together with a meal of that kind, however, is equal to ingesting an antidote together with a poison.

In the following list we list the most frequently consumed vegetables, perhaps it is not complete, but it contains enough vegetables to show how wide a variety we have at our disposal: **spinach, kale, thistles, turnips, beets, cabbage, broccoli, okra, beans, peas, asparagus, green cabbage, lettuce, celery, Chinese cabbage,** etc.! All of these vegetables in their natural state are very tasty and can undoubtedly make up the ingredients in a salad. There are several varieties of lettuce that can be used, even two at a time. In some parts of the country you can buy vegetables such as escarole, endive and others. Cucumber is the delicious addition to a salad, but it can also be eaten on its own.

There is a wide variety of salads, one more or less every season of the year. In fact, it is very important to eat fresh vegetables every day of the year, not just at intervals. **It is advisable not to economize in the consumption of vegetables.** The salads generally served in restaurants and hotels are in quantities too small to meet the needs of those who consume them.

Many people complain that they cannot make much use of that substance commonly called "bran." Dr. Kellogg, years ago, stated that the material generally referred to as "bran" (fiber), should instead be called "bulk". The fact is that the small amount of undigestible cellulose present in these foods, is not raw. On the contrary, it appears soft and full of water. In fact, extracting all the water contained in the vegetable, you would immediately notice that the amount of mass that previously formed its whole, is greatly reduced. So, the fact that vegetables contain too much "fiber" is not based on any concrete evidence. **When vegetables and fruits are cut into small pieces, ground, chopped, grated, left in contact with the oxygen of the air, much of their nutritive value is lost through oxidation. The longer they are left in contact with air after being cut, the greater the loss of nutritional value appears.** During oxidation, the loss of certain vitamins is particularly rapid. Such habits are permitted only for those persons who, having lost their teeth, appear unable to chew whole foods. In these cases, food should be given immediately after preparation in order to limit oxidation and consequently the loss of nutritional value.

The dressings added to salads, in themselves, are not incompatible with them, however, they interfere with the digestion of other foods. The acids contained in condiments damage the digestion of starches and proteins. Oils damage the digestion of proteins. Cream, whether sweet or sour, added to salads, interferes in the digestion of proteins. Sugars inhibit the digestion of proteins. Therefore, while there is no serious reason why oil or cream should not be added to a salad to be eaten with a starchy meal, it should not be done in the case of a salad to be eaten with a protein meal. In both cases, **lemon and vinegar should be avoided. There is no objection to adding lemon or oil, or both, to a salad if it is the only food in the meal.**

The acid contained in tomatoes interferes in the digestion of both proteins and starches. Therefore, it is advisable to eliminate tomatoes from salads in case you consume these types of foods. In the case of cheese, nuts and avocados, which contain oils that inhibit the digestion of proteins longer than acids on starches, tomatoes can be added. Again with these foods the use of lemon or oil is not discouraged. With other proteins the rule applies that "acids and proteins should not be eaten together, but in separate meals."

In general, **I prefer an unseasoned salad, made up of whole vegetables,** i.e. not chopped and shredded. Rather than cutting the tomato into slices, leave it whole in the middle of the salad, arranging the leaves artistically in a circle. The vitamin C in tomatoes is quickly destroyed by oxidation when they are cut into small pieces. **The leaves of the lettuce** should be **left whole**. If a head of lettuce is used, leave it in halves or quarters, depending on the size. A large amount of lettuce should always be part of the salad. **If cucumbers are used, they should be left whole if small, or cut in half if large.** Smaller cucumbers are the tastiest and are not bitter. **Celery should be served whole,** rather than shredded. **Carrots should not be grated.**

The best way to prepare a salad is to serve it simply. Those salads consisting of dozens of ingredients are far from ideal. **Three or four ingredients are sufficient. Lettuce, tomatoes and celery make an excellent salad.** If you want to add a sprig of parsley or bits of red pepper to these for a splash of color, you can easily do so. **Celery, lettuce and cucumber** make up an equally excellent salad. **Romaine lettuce, tender okra and spinach make up** a very tasty salad. **Cabbage, tomato and fresh peas** make up another excellent tasting salad. In fact, there is no limit to the variety and combinations of salads you can form, each rich in minerals and vitamins.

It is vital to feed daily salads to growing children. In fact, salad is more important for children than for adults, although it is also important for adults. Children should be accustomed to eating a salad daily from an early age so that they develop a consistent liking for this food and continue to eat it for the rest of their lives. This is much more useful in the child's diet than any other preparation from the pharmacy, **such as cod liver oil,** mineral or vitamin pills, etc. **Salads are, moreover, richer sources of calcium than milk**, especially nowadays when it is practically impossible to consume milk which has not already been pasteurized. **It cannot be stressed enough that pasteurization alters the calcium salts contained in milk to the point that they are unusable by the child.** I want to close this chapter, therefore, by stating that: *"in our diet nothing can replace fresh vegetables".*

CHAPTER 9 - DIETARY PATTERN FOR A WEEK

All the menus proposed in this book are simply guides intended to help the reader understand the fundamental principles of food combinations in short, to help him formulate his own menu. I am convinced that it is more important to know how to plan one's menu than to have a book containing three meals a day for every day of the year. The person who understands the system of combining foods and who is able to combine his own menu will never find himself in difficulty in preparing his meals. He can always improvise a menu from the foods he has on hand.

However, the same foods may not always be available in every country. A food that is common in one country in a particular season may be common in another in a different season. The availability of foods varies with the season, climate, altitude, land, and ease of market. Anyone who knows how to combine their foods will be able to take advantage of the foods available to them to establish their menu. On the other hand, those who cannot do without a manual-guide and do not know how to combine foods, may find themselves in difficulty when they discover that the foods listed on the menu for that day are not available: they are, in short, in trouble. What unfortunately happens in these circumstances is that the person chooses the easiest way to solve the problem, and that is to eat without criteria. At the home of a friend or relative, the manual cannot be followed scrupulously; knowing, instead, how to combine foods, you can choose compatible combinations of those you put on the table.

Learn the principles governing food combinations in such a way that you can apply them correctly in all circumstances. A child may be able to carefully follow a list; an intelligent adult should learn the concepts and try to apply them. Once this has been achieved, after practicing correct food combinations at home, the habit becomes automatic and much concentration is no longer needed. Above all, one does not have to become manic about this practice. One must eat and end it there. You must leave your friends free to eat as they wish, without starting a discussion on dietetics every time.

The following two-week scheme is intended to demonstrate the proper way to combine foods during the various seasons of the year. The pattern for the first week covers spring and summer. The one for the second, fall and winter. Use them only as a guide and learn to prepare the menus yourself.

9.1 Spring and summer menus

BREAKFAST	LUNCH	DINNER
	SUNDAY	
Watermelon	Salad	Salad
	Thistles	Green beans
	Yellow pumpkin	Gombo
	Potatoes	Walnuts
	MONDAY	
Peaches	Salad	Salad
Cherries	Beets	Spinach
Apricots	Carrots	Cabbage
	Baked beans	Cheese flakes
	TUESDAY	
Cantaloupe melon	Salad	Salad
	Gombo	Broccoli
	Green pumpkin	Fresh corn
	Artichokes	Avocado
	WEDNESDAY	
Berries with cream without sugar)	Salad	Salad
	Cauliflower	Green pumpkin
	Gombo	Turnips
	Brown rice	Lamb chops
	THURSDAY	
Nectarines	Salad	Salad

Apricots	Green cabbage	Beetroot
Plums	Carrots	Green beans
	Sweet potatoes	Walnuts
	FRIDAY	
Watermelon	Salad	Salad
	Baked aubergines	Yellow pumpkin
	Thistles	Spinach
	Wholemeal bread	Eggs
	SATURDAY	
Bananas	Salad	Salad
Cherries	Beans	Kohlrabi
A glass of sour milk	Gombo	Broccoli
	Potatoes	Soybean sprouts

9.2 Menus for autumn and winter

	SUNDAY	
Grapes	Salad	Salad
Bananas	Cabbage	Spinach
Dates	Asparagus	Yellow pumpkin
	Caladum Roots	Baked beans
	MONDAY	
Khaki	Salad	Salad
Pears	Kohlrabi	Brussels sprouts
Grapes	Cauliflower	Green beans
	Sweet potatoes	Walnuts
	TUESDAY	
Apples	Salad	Salad
Grapes	Turnips	Cabbage

Dried figs	Gombo	Yellow pumpkin
	Brown rice	**Avocado**
	WEDNESDAY	
Pears	Salad	Salad
Khaki	Broccoli	Gombo
Bananas	Green beans	Spinach
A glass of sour milk	Potatoes	**Pine nuts**
	THURSDAY	
Papaya	Salad	Salad
Oranges	Carrots	Thistles
	Spinach	Yellow pumpkin
	Boiled Caladium roots	Whole cheese
	FRIDAY	
Khaki	Salad	Salad
Grapes	Green pumpkin	Red cabbage
Dates	Parsnips	Green beans
	Wholemeal bread	Sunflower seeds
	SATURDAY	
Grapefruit	Salad	Salad
	Fresh peas	Spinach
	Kohlrabi	Boiled onions
	Coconut	Lamb chops
	SUNDAY	
Melon	Salad	Salad
	Green beans	Baked aubergines
	Vegetable stock	Kohlrabi
	Sweet potatoes	Eggs

CHAPTER 10 - HOW TO CURE INDIGESTION

The importance of good digestion cannot be underestimated. On the efficiency of the digestive process depends the preparation of the raw materials of nutrition; hence, on good digestion, depends, to a great extent, the well-being of the body. There is no such thing as good nutrition without good digestion. Even the best diet fails in its purpose when the digestive process does not perform well the task of preparing the substances to be used.

Poor digestion cannot supply the materials with which to produce a rich blood; from this it will follow that the tissues will not be properly nourished, that the general health will suffer, and that the constitution will deteriorate. It is very important to remember that the normal process of blood production depends upon the preparation of the materials which serve that purpose, in the digestive tract. Good digestion, therefore, means a normal turnover of tissues throughout the body. Better digestion gives, as a result, a general improvement in all vital functions. Many and immense are the benefits that flow from improved digestion.

Indigestion is the precursor, not the cause, of many of the most serious diseases of man. But every impairment of function, becomes a secondary source of causes, and the poisoning which results from indigestion increases the causes of suffering which add to the primary ones. By preventing indigestion, one keeps healthy; when indigestion is cured, health returns.

An immense variety of disorders and symptoms accompany the progressive deterioration of the digestive function: gas, acid eruptions, a sense of discomfort in the abdomen which gradually turns into pain, sleepless and restless nights, tongue covered with a patina in the morning, anorexia, constipation, foul-smelling stools, nervousness, etc. This is not, however, a complete list of symptoms that accompany indigestion.

If we reflect for a moment on the enormous quantities of digestives (Alka-Seltzer, Bromo-Seltzer, Milk of Magnesia, etc.) consumed by the American population in an attempt to nullify the disorders caused by acid fermentation and gas in the digestive tract, we come to the conclusion that we are a people who suffer from indigestion. Discomfort after meals is extremely common and no one seems able to provide more than a temporary remedy for it. It is sad to admit that so-called "medical science" can do nothing valuable and constructive in a simple functional condition of this nature.

In addition to the drugs generally used to relieve ailments, there are other ways to "aid digestion". Pepsin is perhaps the best known method. It was once claimed that chewing American gum facilitated digestion. This, and other similar types of "aids," are frauds. They do not facilitate digestion at all. They do not improve the functional capacity of the digestive organs at all, nor do they remove the causes of damage. On the contrary, the continued use of these substances further damages the digestive capabilities.

The use of "digestives" and palliatives diverts the attention of the sick from the real solution to their problems and obscures the truths about health and illness and the ways to restore good health. I am continually surprised to find that mankind has always trusted such remedies, all of which are flimsy. **Even fools should learn from repeated mistakes.**

A concept often expressed by medical authorities is that if two foods can be digested "separately," they must also be digested together. They extend this principle to the entire menu: if this item is digestible separately, it can also be digested when eaten together with twenty-one other dishes.

Within limits, this view is true, otherwise the common man would die from lack of food. Instead of dying, he thrives, even grows fat by the use of conventional diets which are nothing but indiscriminate mixtures of the most disparate substances. That the digestion is no longer regular is shown, however, by gas, acid eructations, disorders, **malodorous stools, and the presence in these of large quantities of undigested food. Indeed, at least half of the food consumed by these persons is expelled without being digested.**

It is usually asserted that food may be introduced into the digestive tract in the most disordered manner, in every possible combination, and in the quantity desired by the individual, and that, in spite of this, digestion may be good. This concept is not based on physiological principles, but on the determination of physicians not to disturb the common habits of the people. Every student of physiology knows perfectly well that the enzymes of digestion possess definite limitations, and that, in order to digest different kinds of food, the secretion of different gastric juices is necessary. These limitations must be respected.

The fact is that millions of Americans first feed themselves in the indiscriminate and reckless manner which the medical profession endorses, and then, after each meal, suffer from indigestion. The fantastic profits made each year from the sale of **various digestives such as Alka-Seltzer, Diger-Seltz, etc., prescribed by doctors**, and the unlimited use of substances, such as bicarbonate of soda to try to relieve ailments, seem to be meaningless. Perhaps, as doctors claim, digestion in those cases is efficient. Or, perhaps, does it mean that the complete elimination of such symptoms and ailments would bring too marked a decline in earnings?

To the objection against the consumption of milk together with meat, such persons reply that milk is regularly used together with certain meats, such as crabs, oysters, etc., without causing death by intoxication. The notion enclosed in these words, is that if a thing is done out of habit, it must of necessity be a good thing. Man has never, in the whole course of history, adopted harmful habits. The only healthy thing for a man to do is to eat, drink, and smoke, without paying attention to his health until it fails, at which point he can always go to a doctor and have pills or injections prescribed. If people are accustomed to consume milk together with meat at the same meal, this habit must not be broken, even if it causes discomfort.

Those who consume foods in a disordered manner can learn to combine them according to rules based on the physiology of digestion, avoiding indigestion, malodorous stools, gas and the disorders that usually accompany conventional diets. Every physician can try this on himself and realize it. The fact that physicians, believing themselves to be "men of science" who have espoused "the scientific method" and refuse to test this question, shows their prejudices on the subject. They will, however, reject the "scientific method" if and when there are reasons to think that the results of an experiment may in some way compromise their own and others' habits. Experiments may prove them wrong.

Every student of dietetics knows that the present habits of Americans of combining together the most disparate foods are certainly not those which once existed. **If we take a look at the eating habits of the past, we find them to be very simple.** We also know that a simple diet provides better digestion. If we observe the eating habits of animals inferior to us, we find the greatest simplicity. In fact, they generally tend to eat only one food per meal. It would probably be impossible to force an ape to eat a meal of seven courses or even twenty-one.

Today, we are faced with two concomitant facts, linked together as cause - effect. As fact number one, we have the mixture at every meal of a great variety of foods. As fact number two we have indigestion, accompanied by the taking of medicines intended to alleviate the disorders connected with it. Now, if it can be shown that simple meals are those which are most easily digested and do not cause indigestion, while complex mixtures, regularly eaten cause it, we are confronted with a number of facts which should not be overlooked.

There is an old proverb that says, "it's actions, not words that count". I would like to explain to my readers that the proof of the value of properly combined foods lies in consuming those combinations that comply with the rules we have previously formulated. If such meals put an end to indigestion, it means that they are correct. Of course, food combinations that do not cause indigestion are to be preferred to those that do. It is certainly better to digest food than to resort to medication. Medicines provide temporary relief from the complaints relating to indigestion, but encourage the habits that cause it, producing harm. "There is none so deaf as those who will not hear," says an old proverb. **Intelligent people who close their eyes to the physiological and food-combination evidence guarantee themselves unnecessary discomfort and suffering.**

It is obvious that if you want to put an end to indigestion, you have to adopt radically different eating habits. There is no advantage in enriching the manufacturers and distributors of medicines. Such people make millions from selling products that only make the situation worse. Natural Hygiene offers people **a real way to end the suffering and enslavement to wrong traditions.** Good digestion should be a normal occurrence and if indigestion occurs, it means that the related capabilities are reduced. After considering the effects of an unfavorable environment, one must attribute much of man's suffering to his departure, ignorant as he may be, from the organic laws of life. Health can be preserved only by careful observation of all the laws of life in their combinations.

The digestive process is undoubtedly more efficient when food is consumed in a calm and peaceful state of mind, as opposed to a state of psychological agitation. That is how much the digestive process is influenced by the conduct of the individual after eating, in relation to rest or work! Rest, after eating, is indispensable for good digestion. No one can digest food properly if, out of haste, he does not take care of chewing or if after eating he runs back to work.

When one lives at such a pace, as is often the case in large cities, where everything, including eating, must be consumed quickly, when the jaws cannot chew fast enough and the food is swallowed, chewed only halfway; **when the individual immediately rushes to work without a moment's rest for mind and body, and this, day after day, year after year, to the limit of human endurance, the nemesis of outraged nature takes its toll.** The human capacity to lead such a life is not unlimited, but varies according to the constitutional aspects of different individuals. The strongest will outlast the weakest, but **sooner or later, even the most robust will succumb** to the deteriorating effects of such a life.

When, for either reason, the human constitution is impaired with consequent impairment of vitality, the first symptom of general depression is debilitation of the digestive powers.

We must consider, if only for a moment, the many influences that certainly diminish man's bodily vigor in order to realize how, in modern society, everyone is more or less debilitated. We may divide these influences into sins of commission and sins of omission. Sins **of omission** are those due to ignorance of the laws of nature or to willful neglect, or both. Sins of **commission,** on the other hand, are those in which the laws of nature are not only deliberately ignored, but this happens for the purpose of profit or pleasure. Debilitating influences can also be divided into those caused by necessity or struggle for survival, (in a socio-economic environment in which man possesses no power of control), and those that are causal or even deliberately sought after. The hardships of misery and poverty of the lower classes appear equal to the dissipation and debilitating luxuries of the higher classes. **Speculation, gambling and excitement of all kinds appear to be the most harmful factors to the nervous system.** However, whether from the physical or mental fatigue of the worker, or from the suicidal mania of the arrived man, or from other factors still, the result is the same.

With the constant violation of the laws of nature, that is, with the repetition of debilitating activities, the energies of the organism are diminished, and this causes a progressive weakening of the nerves which is not always immediately recognized. The result is a prostration in mental and physical abilities and a general degradation of the subject.

When, as a result of continued neglect of the laws of life, the constitutional capacities appear weakened, not only does the excretory function appear greatly weakened, resulting in toxaemia (the state of poisoning which results from the retention of waste substances), but the digestive and assimilative capacities also appear impoverished, and the degree of nutrition of the body is equal to the level of constitutional weakening. This causes indigestion and all consequent disorders. In an individual so debilitated, a change in diet will not restore health unless the causes which have caused the state of emaciation are removed and the body is allowed a period of rest which will help it to re-establish its natural functional activities. It should, therefore, appear obvious that if the ability to digest and assimilate food is not improved, all efforts to restore the individual to health will be in vain. It is even more futile to try to restore the digestive abilities by the use of **medicines** - tonics, astringents, mineral acids, iron preparations, etc., as these further damage the system. - as these **further damage the weakened digestive system.**

Replacing one source of weakening with another is not a rational procedure. To undergo rest and at the same time to undertake a series of palliative treatments: baths, massages, electrical applications, enemas, colon irrigations, etc., will not serve to restore good health. Remember that learning to live according to the laws of life will serve to free you forever from ailments and suffering.

Only by living within the limits of physiological and biological laws will it be possible to transform the cry of pain that rises from the earth today into a joyful song.

The intelligent person, having ascertained the numerous diseases which arise from violations of the most natural dietary laws of life, will at once recognize **the first step to be taken in the attempt to restore health: namely, the return to simplicity and the strictest obedience to the rules which he had hitherto ne-**

glected. He who wishes to restore his health must regain habits of life that conform as closely as possible to the laws of nature.

Is it possible to treat a person who is seeking health differently? Is it possible to conceive of a person in search of health being "cured" with medicines, serums, vaccines or even surgery? It is impossible, unless, of course, one forgets the physiological principles that govern human life.

In the first place it is necessary that the nervous system, already overworked by work, abuse, stimulation (irritation), excesses of various kinds, etc., be put to rest. So I would recommend a preliminary period of complete detachment from all physical and mental activities and duties that absorb most of the nervous resources. This is the "condicio sine qua non" of recovery.

It is necessary, first of all, for the debilitated individual to rest, mentally and physically.

The physiological importance of mental rest on the performance of the digestive functions explains the considerable importance we have given to the practice of nervous rest. Mental rest is best guaranteed by a detachment from the workplace, from the 'polluted' atmosphere of the cities, from the noise, by moving to the peace of the countryside, in a place with varied and picturesque scenery, with clean air, where the individual can find relaxation, rejoice in nature and enjoy its beneficial rays of the sun.

Such arguments highlight that over time, medication does nothing to solve the problem. On the contrary, they worsen the situation. The progressive deterioration of functions is not only due to the deleterious effect of medicines, but also to neglect of the causes. It is useless to think of "curing" the disease without removing the causes that caused it.

Everyone has access to the two "paths" of life One leads to health, strength, happiness and longevity; it gives us the crown of honour, of the richest and most abundant life. The other leads to sickness, weakness, unhappiness and premature death. It bestows upon us the crown of dishonor, sorrow, and a meaningless life. Which path do you want to follow? The choice is yours: no one can decide for you. Law and order do not respect people and everyone will be rewarded or penalized according to the life he chooses. Do you lead a dissipated life, wasting time and money to satisfy appetites that exceed the needs of a normal life? What are your habits? Are they so wholesome that they benefit you? Do you abuse gambling or perverse habits? Are you sure that your way of life, your physical and mental practices, are consistent with the laws of life? Remember that the best use of body and mind is the one that provides happiness and progress.

The problem cannot be dealt with unilaterally. We are talking about a problem that has developed as a result of a multitude of factors and cannot be solved by eliminating just a few of them. **It is not enough to change just one debilitating habit. All of them must be discontinued immediately** if a good state of health is to be achieved.

In the same way that in restoring the functional capacity of a weak organism the first step is the interruption of debilitating habits, so the second is the rational use of properly combined materials, and of the influences which form the Hygienic System. After the total removal of the causes of weakening, sleep, rest, proper nutrition, exercise, clean air, pure water, sunshine, and sound moral and mental habits are indispensable to the attainment of integrity and full efficiency of function.

When, with Hygienic practices, the body is freed from toxic accumulations, the nervous energy returns to normal, the process of elimination is restarted and so are the digestive and assimilative abilities; the body gradually returns to health. Until this point is reached, no diet can solve the problem. Non-observance of these rules may lead to the onset of acute and chronic diseases sometimes even fatal, so that abrupt limitations in diets are inefficient.

Hygienic factors are not of great importance in local treatment, but they certainly have a beneficial effect upon the organism as a whole. Thus, food does not have value in localized situations, but in relation to its use by the whole organism. As a basic foundation of the work of a hygienist, we guarantee the full benefit of hygienic practices, as only in this way can the individual regain his or her health. On this basis, the term Natural Hygiene acquires a real and meaningful meaning.

It must be emphasized that food alone, however important it may be, whether in health or disease, is not sufficient to ensure the restoration or maintenance of health. Only if it is physiologically linked to water, exercise, rest, sleep and the other elements of the hygienic system, can it express its value. Rest, more than any other element, appears to be important, even though they are all indispensable; in the natural hygienic system, health is not restored by a single hygienic factor alone, but by the complete utilization of all of them.

I repeat again that, as a scientific fact, it is the whole of the above-mentioned hygienic components, in their harmonious combination, that constitute the material employed by the organism in the recovery of health. Natural or Hygienic care of the sick person, consisting of many interdependent factors, cannot be held responsible if, by neglecting one or more of these elements, the purpose is not achieved.

Physiological rest (fasting) is of great value in all forms of health impairment, but in the case of indigestion it is the only way to provide rest for the fatigued digestive system. During a fast all the organs of the body reduce their activity, so they rest. The exception is the excretory organs, which increase their activity: therefore, during a fast, the body can get rid of accumulations of toxic substances. The combinations of mental, physical and physiological rest together constitute the ideal means of promoting elimination.

Fasting should not be practiced at home, a place of distractions, disturbances, and responsibilities, where friends and relatives may be averse. It should be undertaken in a Hygienic clinic under the guidance of an expert. In the Hygienic clinic, the individual is in a physical and mental position that makes it easier, not only to fast, but also to break bad habits. Here he can develop and cultivate better habits. Indeed, it is best that he should remain there until the new habits have become firm points in his life. This is of vital importance for the continued progress of health, once it has been regained.

Let's not forget that physical well-being, once lost, can only be regained through a laborious process in which the individual plays the main role: that is, to systematically practice healthy habits until the point of reaching the goal.

APPENDIX

FEEDING RAW FOODS

There are two ways to approach the subject of nutrition. Hygienists use the biological approach. It consists in determining man's place in nature to the point where his dietary character is involved. Is man a carnivore, a herbivore, an omnivore, a saprophyte, or a fruitarian? Once you have determined his true classification you can determine the best resources of human food.

Having done so, we can confidently eat those raw, unrefined, **raw, unseasoned, unsalted and unsophisticated foods** straight from their true nature and be sure to secure adequate nutrition without worrying about calories, protein or vitamins. Why should man study the chemistry of food to try to feed himself more than a horse or an elephant should?

The other approach is the biochemical approach. This approach chemically analyzes the human body and its excreta as well as the foods that man eats. From all this one tries to find and derive diets in the same way as the chemist. The biochemist is an egomaniac who believes that he can deal with the chemistry of life. He believes that he can make the body do what he wants. He is the one who invents all the mineral concentrates, vitamin supplements, amino acid additives, etc., that he can make the body do what he wants. Instead of giving bananas or dates or persimmons, refined sugar is given and then the supplements are given.

I personally believe that the biological approach is the only true method of achieving proper nutrition and eliminating the causes of disease. We don't cure disease through proper nutrition, we prevent it.

Man is classified as a frugivore. **His diet should consist of fruits, vine fruits (vegetables), nuts, and seeds and they should be eaten in a raw state as much as possible.** The more natural our foods are and their unprocessed state, the better off we are. The natural "affinity" that exists between the needs of our cells and the nutritional elements of natural foods provides us with an unerring guarantee that they provide us with salts, vitamins and other elements from natural foods. **All "real" foods taste much better raw than cooked.**Cooked foods, without seasoning, are flat and bland to the palate, as well as less nutritious.

Ripe fruits, vegetables, nuts, and seeds are "made" by nature. When we cook them we destroy them. We take away their enzymes and vitamins and turn organic minerals into inorganic minerals.

For most people, the digestibility of food is not improved by cooking and the value of food is reduced.

A raw food diet initiates the cleansing operation of the body and may result in headaches or symptoms of uric acid poisoning the body. Gas may occur in the stomach in the first few days. You may feel tired, but all this proves is that there were poisons in your body that needed to be expelled. After your body is clean you will feel good and full of energy.

Why does a raw food diet cause this? First of all because raw vegetables, fruits, nuts and seeds were given to us by nature. All life on earth is completely dependent on the sun. Therefore, vitality is synonymous with solar energy. Humans and animals cannot assimilate everything they need to grow from the sun. Plants take that energy and store it in their roots, fruits and seeds which we then use for human growth. We use plants as an intermediary between the sun and ourselves.

Fresh, raw food constitutes human food, the true resource of life!

Fresh, raw fruits and vegetables possess the highest nutritional value for mankind. It cannot be increased by drying, wilting, storage, fermentation or preservation. Its nutritive value is reduced by process of any kind.

What criteria should we use when selecting raw foods?
1. Can foods be eaten in their natural state?
2. Does food introduce harmful substances into our food system?
3. Is the food delicious, tasty? Can it be eaten with gusto in its natural state?
4. Is the food easy for digestion and assimilation?
5. Does food contribute to a wide range of nutrition? Does food possess great biological value for us?
6. Is the food acid-causing in the metabolic reaction? Is it alkaline in metabolic reaction?

7. Is the food cheap?

8. Is the food accessible in its natural state throughout the year?

Keep your body pure. Don't tease it with anything. And keep in mind, that nothing will fill you up except the foods for which we human beings are naturally adapted, and that is fresh ripe fruit, green succulent vegetables, nuts and some seeds, all raw, **all eaten in the freshest possible state, just taken from nature.**

The plant kingdom represents the great farm of the world. We do not need any other resources for our foods. Animal foods are only second-hand products and should be used frugally in times of cold or famine. Processed, lab-derived foods are abominable.

PROTEIN (IMPORTANT, BUT BE CAUTIOUS)

Protein building blocks consist of 21 amino acids. Nine of these have been proven to be essential for the support of life and growth. Proteins containing all the amino acids are called complete or first class. A food that contains a complete protein will support life and growth when used as a protein base in the diet.

It is often stated that the difficulty of obtaining complete protein in a fruitarian diet makes such a diet dangerous. BUT THIS IS NOT TRUE. There is an abundance of foods derived from plants that supply us with complete protein of the highest biological value. Research has shown that the protein in most nuts is of the finest type and contains all the convenient and essential amino acids. Nuts that possess complete protein include butternuts, American walnuts, hazelnuts, Brazil nuts, English walnuts, almonds, pine nuts, coconuts and chestnuts.

To complete, the protein in most nuts is of a rather high biological quality. It has been proven that the protein in walnuts not only provides more nutritional efficiency than that of meat, milk and eggs, but is also much more of a combination of animal proteins.

Coconut globulin represents the best nut protein. McCandish and Weaver found that coconut protein is superior to that of other foods, and they claim that **the coconut meal is of greater value than the soybean meal.** Coconut contains probably one of the best proteins known.

No frugivore should ever have to worry about their protein supplies. Any well-balanced selection of foods should meet the protein needs of the body very well. In fact, it will replenish much better than the diet of omnivores (meat eaters) as it replenishes the protein in just the right amounts.

Overeating protein rich foods is the primary cause of our diseases. One doctor stated that if we don't eat protein for at least 17 hours in the course of a day, we won't get cancer.

It is almost impossible to name at least one food that does not contain protein. They are found in anything that grows. **A banana not only contains about 15% protein (dry weight) but also all the essential amino acids.** Celery contains about 15% protein and lettuce around 20%. So don't get fossilized on the protein issue as you move towards a naturally raw diet.

More than any other dietary factor, excess protein fills the body with toxins. Foods rich in concentrated protein such as eggs, meat, cheese, etc. can cause various types of ailments if eaten in abundance.

What is needed in America these days is not more protein or more amino acids but a genuine return to a natural way of eating.

GLUTTONY AND OVEREATING

A very necessary rule for health is:

EAT ONLY WHEN YOU ARE HUNGRY!

If you eat when your body does not require it you are asking it to do extra and unnecessary work. Overeating leads to obesity, belly-aching, and accumulates putrefying matter that can give rise to a wide variety of diseases.

Therefore, overeating is a cause of illness. Three meals a day plus intervals of "coffee" and croissants is like throwing darts at footballs, and you represent footballs. When something "stings" you get sick.

There has been a lot of talk about how a "hearty breakfast gets your day off to a good start". Well, indeed it does ... at least for those people who sell you all the things you eat for breakfast ... People who make cold cereal, collect eggs and squeeze oranges make a fortune. Certainly their day starts well, but at your expense.

The sole purpose of eating is to nourish the body and eating should be a pleasurable experience. Thousands of factories are amassing millions of dollars by appealing to the "pleasure of eating." It seems that the idea of nourishing our bodies is less important than the pleasure of eating. Foods that could be perfect are being ground, chopped, cooked, crushed, grated, flavored, fried, baked, salted, sugared, preserved, processed, packaged, advertised and SOLD to us in a new form and with a nice package and at a high price.

Chips, ice cream, pizza, candy and a million other food items are designated to make money coming from your wallet and appealing to your TASTE AND ... IT WORKS. Witness all the "tasty" products that appear on television that are nothing more than warnings that television manages to give in an attempt to alleviate all the problems you have. This adds filth on top of filth. It is just plain silly.

Most of these "refined" foods are lacking in water so there is a tendency to overeat or become a glutton. The opposite happens when you eat raw foods containing enough water because good food fills you up before you can eat too much. With high food prices, it's silly to spend our money trying to fill ourselves up with foods we don't absolutely need. The greatest sin of Americans is overeating.

A tendency to overeat is caused by choosing too many foods at one meal. How many times (in the past) have I loaded my stomach, plate after plate, because of the variety and also because I could have everything I wanted for the price of one food. **It is amazing how I can satisfy myself with a single food or at most two and rarely get to four or five.** You too can enjoy foods and achieve superlative health.

Don't confuse hunger with appetite. Hunger is "a feeling that makes a person want to eat". Appetite is a "feeling that causes a person to want to eat a food PARTICULARLY".

Hunger makes a rabbit want food, but his appetite advises him to eat grass. It is the same for the wolf, but to him his appetite suggests eating the rabbit. They both want to eat what their palate seeks.

Nature makes our food tasty so that we have to eat it. However, man has learned to "make fun of mother nature" and is busy producing endless tasty foods that are not as nutritious as real natural foods. Currently, mother nature is never mocked. We are.

Nowadays, shape, color, smell, temperature, etc. are all about palatability and scientists think they can make us eat even powder if they make it taste good. What they do instead is take good food and make it mush even if they make it look desirable. At this point it is natural that we develop a perverse taste.

Discarded and diner foods have a certain attractiveness, tastiness, palatability. How many people do you know who might choose a fresh salad over a bowl of banana with a heap of ice cream and cream and all made more attractive by the red cherry at the top? Compare the fruit and vegetable shops in your country with those selling ice cream and other "delicacies" and you will have the answer. Many people will definitely vote for ice cream, but all is not lost. Many restaurants are now discovering the importance of salad and people are amazed at the incredible flavor of this food.

I know now that I can eat and rejoice in what I feel is best for my body and I am no longer a slave to my appetite. I know that my taste and appetites were formed in my childhood and I understand that I can change those tastes and appetites. I am no longer tempted by salty, sugary and refined foods. I will never again use the excuse that "the devil made me eat it!"

EAT ONLY TWO MEALS A DAY

Eating three meals a day is an invention of modern man that has come about only in the past hundred years. The fashion for coffee breaks, snacks and naps have only come to light in the last few decades.

Appetite means "strong desire." If we have an appetite for food we also have a strong desire for eating. Being a slave to appetites leads to being a glutton.

Television, newspaper and radio constantly bombard us with warnings about "good things to eat". Virtually any new cookbook released on the market is an instant hit. All of this has led us to be addicted to food, creating appetites that we cannot control.

However ALL OF THESE USELESSNESSES ... can be stopped when you finally realize that it all makes no sense. People are getting rich by selling products that fill our mouths. We actually use foods as entertainment. When we consume what we call "breakfast", and usually from 6.00 A.M. to 9.00 P.M. we are breaking our fast from dinner during the night.

If you have to eat something early in the morning, despite what you read below, then eat one fruit at a time such as melon, orange, grapes, plums, pears, apples, or other fruits. This will give your body as little shock as possible and you will get the most out of your food. Don't feel guilty if you only eat one fruit for breakfast. Later, you can develop your eating habits more fully than your body requires.

To understand "why" we should only eat two meals a day we need to understand "our body's biological clock".

During the night of rest and sleep, your body is assimilating the previous day's food and loading up on nervous energy. When you get up in the morning your body has no need for food as there is no lack of energy. It is in fact, already charged and ready to go. In this first cycle of the day food should normally be repulsive to you. Your body should feel "recovered" after a good night's rest and sleep and is eager to be engaged in some activity other than eating. You should have an interest in "doing something".

The body undergoes three distinct phases in each 24-hour period.

1. Food Appropriation. This phase does not begin until you are hungry. This habitually happens around noon when you have started to run out of your glycogen resources through activity. You need to eat during midday and dinner.

2. Food Assimilation. This phase begins late in the evening and goes on until the early hours of the morning. During this time of rest and sleep, the body performs its homework.

3. Elimination of the body's metabolic waste and ingested toxic materials. This phase usually begins in the very early hours of the morning and lasts until noon. Our appetite and digestive system drops (?) during these hours. Psychologically we may need food, but there is no physiological demand for it. We would never really be hungry. If we eat during this phase, the energies directed toward cleansing the body will have to be redirected again toward digestion. It is always a shock to the body to interrupt its biological alarm clock. When we eat breakfast we interfere with the normal operations of the body.

In spite of everything said by the breakfast makers YOUR BODY DOES NOT NEED well-fed breakfasts. And here's another myth busted!

DIETARY RULES (SUMMARY)

Some of these rules about nutrition are more fully explained somewhere else rather than here.

RULE 1: Eat only when you are hungry. Do not confuse hunger with appetite. The mouth and throat will tell the brain when they need food. Our bellies may give false alarms until we get them used to accepting what they need and when we no longer become dependent on food.
How many times as soon as we get up from the table do we go back to rummaging in the fridge? How many times, before going to bed, do we open the cupboard or the doorframe to look for something to put under our teeth? If we eat a good dinner we won't be hungry until the next morning ... and usually after noon.

RULE 2: Eat only when free from emotional stress. When you eat you should be calm, relaxed, worry-free, unhurried and in a joyful state of mind. Never eat when you are sick, tired, sore, angry, frustrated or upset.

RULE 3: Do not drink immediately before, during or after meals.

RULE 4: Eat only foods that go along with you. They should be delicious foods that are a pleasure to eat. If the food you eat does not taste good to you then don't eat it, as your digestive juices will not flow.

RULE 5: Eat only foods that are natural to the human diet. Man is primarily a frugivore. This means that he is constitutionally suited to a diet of fruits, succulent vegetables, green leaves, nuts and seeds. Not all fruits or all vegetables or green leaves but a narrow range in relation to all things that grow.

RULE 6: Chew your food carefully.

RULE 7: **Don**'t overfeed and ... don't underfeed. There are two forms of malnutrition. It is one thing to eat too much of a certain food and another to eat too little of it. Eating food beyond our digestive capabilities makes no sense at all as it only becomes material for bacterial decomposition. The body wastes energy refining food that we don't need. It is better to eat as little as you can and not the other way around.

RULE 8 : Eat your foods in compatible combinations. Variety is the spice of gluttony.

RULE 9 : Rest after eating. Do not engage in rigorous exercises or activities. If you exercise just before the meal, your appetite will decrease but it will also shut down your digestive power. So rest and relax a little even before eating.

RULE 10 : Take at least **a five-hour break between meals.** Two meals a day, one at noon and one at dinner is ideal. Eating to live requires strangely little food and we can survive on one good meal a day.

RULE 11 : Eat foods at room temperature or just lukewarm or cold. Hot foods destroy digestive enzymes and have none of their own. Hot foods destroy living cells and cause irritation, inflammation, ulceration and fibrillation. Cold foods inhibit enzyme activity and slow down the digestive process. Therefore, eat foods at a room temperature.

RULE 12 : Eat only in pleasant environments and among equally pleasant people. Uncomfortable environments and the same kind of people create as much discomfort in the stomach. Digestion is suspended in disconcerting circumstances.

RULE 13 : Eat only fresh foods in their natural state. When you eat, these foods will increase the white cells. Foods cooked to 120-190 degrees have their enzymes destroyed and will increase cells, but if they are eaten with some raw foods the number of white cells remains the same. Foods cooked to a higher degree than 190 will increase white cells when eaten, and so will they when eaten with raw foods.

RULE 14 : Eat only foods that are pleasant and tasty and as nature intended. Nutrition is diminished or destroyed in foods that are cooked, refined, mixed, or improperly combined.

RULE 15 : Eat at least 80% of food that is alkaline in metabolic reactions. Cooked foods cause a harmful acid that in their natural state they would not cause.

Nuts and legumes are almost the only foods that produce an acidic end product, but if you eat them after a large salad the acid will disappear.

RULE 16 : Eat meat, eggs, milk, or any other animal food seldom and only in case of very cold weather or famine. All animal products form acid in the human food system. It is possible to be perfectly healthy without eating animal products.

RULE 17 : Bread, as a "life support", should be consumed moderately. **Sprouted wheat constitutes a very nutritious food and is considered more of a vegetable than a grain. Sprouts of many species are delicious and healthy. By eating three tablespoons of wheat sprouts every day with a salad** you will have quite good nutrition.

Whole wheat bread can be a good food, but cooking destroys some of the nutrients. The biggest problem with eating bread is the fact that we generally eat this highly starchy food with foods full of sugar or jam. We habitually eat it in the wrong combinations.

Commercial bread contains so many additives and is so processed that it is not really good food. Baking, however, makes the starches in cereals more digestible. It's best **to go easy on grains** if you can, and especially processed grains that are a total waste of time, money and energy when compared to raw foods.

RULE 18 : Never eat condiments. This means no salt, spices or pepper. Stay away from vinegar, sauces, contominos, onions, garlic, mustard etc. They are all irritants. Irritants interfere with digestion and may even interrupt it.

RULE 19 : Do not allow anything other than whole, enjoyable food to enter your body. This means we must reject anything that is not healthy or necessary for our system. It also means complete abstention from coffee, tea, chocolate, water with chlorine and medicines.

Most of the basic causes of disease come from what we put into our bodies. All diseases are caused by toxemia, which is nothing else than the poisoning of cells, tissues and organs.

Toxemia can, in addition, be caused by poor lifestyle habits, as well as poor eating habits.

CHEW YOUR FOOD (CHEW, CHEW AND CHEW)

Food that has been completely shredded by chewing is readily accessible to the digestive juices. Foods that are swallowed in chunks take longer to digest. We can recover much more energy in the digestive process if we consume a little of it by chewing our food carefully.

Swallowing food without chewing it leads to overeating, rushed eating and all the problems that come with it. When you eat, take a bite, chew it carefully and swallow it before you put another one in your mouth.

Starches and sugars that are thrown down with water, coffee or soda will surely ferment, giving rise to acidity that will make life unpleasant. Starches and sugars that are not chewed carefully and inhaled into the mouth before swallowing will cause digestive problems.

Your tongue plays an important function. It telegraphs to the stomach what kind of food is going to be sent to it, and it prepares the proper acid or alkaline secretion capable of keeping the digestive work going. As the food is chewed and salted the tongue is busy taking messages to send them to the stomach. If it sends the message that some protein is coming, the juices are prepared. If immediately after these it sends the message that a large amount of starch is coming then a great deal of confusion happens in the stomach as acid and alkaline secretions meet.

Proteins do not require as much chewing as starches and sugars because the saliva in the mouth primarily begins the digestive process for starches and sugars only.

There are some side effects from chewing our foods. It cleans our teeth. It exercises the muscles of our head and gives our face a certain tone rather than a whale-like appearance. Lack of chewing causes opposite effects.

FORGET THE SALT

The most important thing we do is eat. Food is much more important for nutritional value than for the joy of eating. From raw foods we can get all the proteins, carbohydrates, fats, vitamins, minerals and other nutrients we need to live. However, all foods are not equal. Some of the foods we eat replenish nutrients in equal proportions while others do not. Some foods can build a strong body while others can produce toxemia which then produces disease. There is an ugly truth in the statement, "You are what you eat."

If you are suffering from toxemia and poor health you can be sure that you have eaten the wrong combination of foods. On the other hand, if you have vibrant health, great strength, and abundant energy you have definitely applied a good combination.

The role of SALT in our modern life is pernicious. It appears in practically everything we eat or place it on raw foods. The body, therefore, receives a heavy load of salt in its inorganic form which is not usable for all forms of animal life.

The chief objection to salt is the fact that it interferes with the normal digestion of food. Pepsin, an enzyme found in the hydrochloric acid of the stomach, is essential for the digestion of proteins. But, when salt is used only half as much pepsin is secreted. Under such a condition the digestion of protein food is incomplete or slow. The results of excessive putrefaction of proteins is in many cases digestive stress.

Salt is primarily the cause of edema (water in the tissues). This represents a defensive action by which the body attempts to keep salt in solution to protect the tissues. It is often stated that salt is essential for life support. However, there is no documentation to prove this point of view. Some entire primitive races do not use salt.

The advice to use salt in hot water comes from the belief that because we sweat a lot, it must be dissolved. In fact, through sweating, which is a part of the excretory system, the body is merely getting rid of the poison ... the salt.

People would not eat salt if the idea of doing so had not been instilled in them. We develop the habit because of the continued presence of the salt shaker on our table. Throw it away. Once salt disappears from the table we no longer feel cramps and become repulsed by its taste.

PURE WATER

How can there be so much misunderstanding about a substance as common as water? We all know that every body needs water, but while some experts say that we need natural mineral water, others say that what we need is water "treated with chlorine and fluoride"; still others say that we should only drink distilled water and still others say that we have no need to drink at all because the water we need comes from the food we eat. As long as you come to the end of this chapter you will determine for yourself what you think is most correct. I do not pretend to state my beliefs in this minimal space, but further information is plausible for those who pursue this interesting subject.

It may surprise you to understand how human beings are not animals that drink natural water. We are much more like desert creatures. Nature did not give us elongated faces with lapping tongues.

You should be pleased to know that if we eat the right foods consisting mainly of ripe fruits, succulent vegetables and appropriately combined nuts, our diet will make up for our water demands.

Yet water from fruits and vegetables is of the purest kind we can receive. Water that is associated with anything else is impure.

But let's see what exactly is the role of water in our body. We don't digest it. It has almost entirely a single function. It is the body's means of transportation. Water in the blood carries nutrients, as well as chemicals and poisons from our digestive tract, lungs and skin. Then, the water in the blood picks up excretions from the cells and transports them to the eliminative organs of the body to excrete them. Our bladder, colon, skin and lungs depend on water to operate.

There are only three inorganic agents from which the body can benefit: oxygen, water and sunlight. Anything else inorganic represents a poison to our body. The body's cells can **only** use **pure water from food or distilled water that is free of inorganic minerals. The cells reject the inorganic and chemical minerals that are found in ordinary water. However, not all of these rejected**

minerals are expelled from the body. Some of them settle in the joints, veins and even in the brain causing problems later on. You may not realize it today, but just wait a little longer!

Those who claim that distilled water removes minerals from the body have never studied the role of the cell or the role of the liver and kidneys. The cell rejects unusable substances and retains its needs. You should only drink when the body requires it through thirst, and **when you drink you should only take one type of water at a time...DISTILLED WATER.**

The human being today is a kind of animal who drinks for his pleasure as well as for his satisfaction. Most of the water we drink contains inorganic metals, chloride, sodium chloride, helium, sulfuric acid, lime, pesticides and other poisons that are harmful to cells.

The human organism cannot use these inorganic minerals and contours. If this were possible we could drink seawater without becoming intoxicated or even dying.

Americans today drink about $26 trillion worth of soda containing caffeine, phosphoric acid, sugar and an incredible number of other poisonous additives that we can't even name. Each year we consume an average of $118 per person to put these chemical concoctions into our bodies and force our bodies to fight against them. Our bodies do not seek out all of these chemical agents and therefore do not use them. Transporting these agents through the circulatory system, heart, and kidneys takes a lot of energy out of your system. Our excretory organs have to work hard to eliminate this "tastes so good" junk. Why don't you grab a nice ripe peach, melon or salad when you are thirsty? You CAN control your appetites. Don't let them control you.

There is no other drink besides fresh water that we can need. Those who pour beer into their stomachs and swallow alcohol are paying for illnesses that will and usually do come in the form of stomach aches and headaches. These so-called illnesses are simply signals by which the body tells us that it has received things it absolutely did not want. It can cause a pain or a fever or diarrhea or vomiting and what is done about it? Instead of eliminating the cause, most people put even more chemicals into their bodies to relieve the pain and gorge themselves on alka seltzer, aspirin or any one of thousands of poisons. You had to get used to beer, alcohol and cigarettes and **you can get used to moving away from such chemicals if you REALLY WANT TO BE HEALTHY.**

If you really want to have a great drink and if you are really thirsty, try drinking "distilled water that flows from stones". Your body will be very grateful.

It is also possible to drink too much water just as it is possible to drink too little. Both of these extremes are harmful. Your body will signal you when it is that you need water.

DON'T DRINK DURING MEALS

NO, NO, AND NO. During a meal of raw foods or well combined foods there is absolutely no need to drink. All the liquid you need will come from the foods you are eating. Even concentrated proteins, from nuts and seeds will get the moisture they need from the vegetables you are eating.

Laboratory tests prove that water leaves the stomach within ten minutes after it is swallowed. If, on the other hand, you drink while you are eating, then the **water will also take away the diluted digestive juices and what is left in the stomach will not be digested perfectly.**

If you feel thirsty you should drink water about fifteen minutes before a meal. If you have eaten and feel thirsty, you can drink water about 30 minutes after a fruit-based meal, two hours after a starch-based meal, and at least four hours after a protein-based meal.

Chewing food carefully to insalivate it with the secretions of the mouth is the first step towards good digestion. If we get into the bad habit of drinking and then cleaning up half-chewed food, we will get into the very bad habit of swallowing huge mouthfuls and we will surely have great digestive problems.

Some times a mouthful of hot food will require a large amount of water to cool the mouth. In this case the body is attacked by the owner and it will rebel by not digesting the food at all.

Hot foods and drinks of the same kind weaken the stomach and take away the power of mechanical action on foods. Weakening the tissues of the stomach through hot drinks or foods creates problems. Extreme heat or cold interferes with the secretion of digestive juices. These juices work best at body temperature.

Iced drinks such as water, lemonade, punch, iced tea, etc. that are often consumed during a meal will slow or delay digestion. The cold temperatures will stop the digestive enzymes which cannot function until body temperature is regained. All this causes thirst and that is why people get thirsty after eating

ice cream. The cold causes a shock and therefore a thirst reaction.

The water in coffee, tea, cocoa, lemonade, etc., not only dilute the digestive juices but also stimulate the appetite and tend to overfeed us. The powerful chemical agents, present in the three drinks just mentioned, act as excitants. The habitual use of these damages the digestion, the kidneys and collapses the nervous system.

Drinking during meals constitutes a bad habit that can be easily eliminated. It is also not about willpower. Simply don't put a cup or glass near your plate while eating. You will learn to love the taste of the deliciousness of fruits and the liquids from fresh vegetables. You will feel your mouth full of tasty liquids. YOU WILL REJOICE IN EATING.

WHAT TO EXPECT FROM DIETARY IMPROVEMENT

Dr Stanley Bass says: <<If I were asked 'what is the area of least understanding in the field of nutrition?' I would be forced to answer 'it is the existing failure to properly understand and interpret the symptoms and changes that follow the initiation of an improved nutritional program'>>.

What is meant by a better nutritional program? It is the replacement of lesser quality foods with those that have more. The closer we get to eating foods with all natural enzymes the closer we will be to having all the amino acids in their best form. The minerals, vitamins, trace elements, carbohydrates and proteins will all be there.

The better the quality of the foods we eat, the better and more perfect our health will be. If we are sick, we will get well sooner if we eat foods properly.

The main rule is as follows: when the quality of food put into the body is better than that of the tissues that make up the body itself, then the body will begin to discard the low grade of materials so as to build new and healthier ones. This is the way nature works.

The body is always trying to build health and will do so unless we interfere by putting poisons into it and sending them to the cells. Nature tells us when we eat wrongly or are putting poisons into our bodies. This condition appears to us in the form of colds, headaches, fevers, or various aches and pains. Illness is the effect of a cause. We avoid the cause to try to avoid the effect (the disease). It is as simple as that.

You may experience symptoms of withdrawal when you begin to eat a better diet. For example, if you are **a coffee drinker** and you suddenly stop drinking coffee, you will probably experience excruciating headaches and a "crash" feeling. This is all caused by the blood criculation trying hard to get the caffeine or theine out of the tissues. These irritants cause pain before they are finally eliminated.

Because you felt better on the old diet you will be tempted to go back on it.

This is all that happens to an addict when he stops using all at once. In fact, an addict always feels better when they can take a dose. Your body, then, used to coffee will probably feel better after getting a "good" cup, but surely when you quit you will feel much better and be healthier.

Some people may feel a little down from 10 days to several weeks. Hang in there, though, because your body is telling you that it is eliminating the waste products that are stored in your tissues. Any sense of weakness you feel is not real weakness. You are simply going through the storm before the quiet.

It is important at this point to stop wasting energy. **Make sure you get enough rest and sleep.** Avoid any kind of stimulant and medicine during this period. Have patience and hope and wait.

Realize that your body is regaining valuable energy to get rid of toxins. **All the poisons from aspirin, sleeping pills and other drugs will be expelled from your body. Along with these you will also lose the piles of fat you have been surrounding yourself with.** In the first phase, the body accentuates the elimination and breakdown of tissues so as to remove the "junk" in them. The body begins its "cleansing" work. It removes, in short, the logs in order to have a better fire.

Waste is eliminated faster than new tissue is formed and therefore you will notice some weight loss. The body will require less food during this period.

The cleansing of the body can take a very long time. It may be that you are eating perfectly and yet still experience symptoms of illness. Those who have abused their bodies much longer and in a much more pronounced way will take longer to reach a state of perfect health. The majority of people find their reactions tolerable and think they will give up their bad habits because of their increased well-being.

Realize, too, that your body is undergoing some rejuvenation and becoming healthier every day as it is eliminating the waste that would most likely have brought pain, illness and much suffering.

Those who suffer the worst manifestations of pain while changing their bad habits for new ones will avoid the worst diseases that could even develop into cancer.

In the final stage health finally arrives, but don't expect it to arrive overnight; it will probably happen in cycles. You may have diarrhea and then feel great, have a cold and then feel great. All of this doesn't happen like flipping a switch.

Soon you'll be telling pretty much everyone that you feel as great as you ever have in all these years. And soon you will experience a great sense of well-being. Before too long you will reach a natural state of mind, and great joy will spread through those who obey the laws of life.

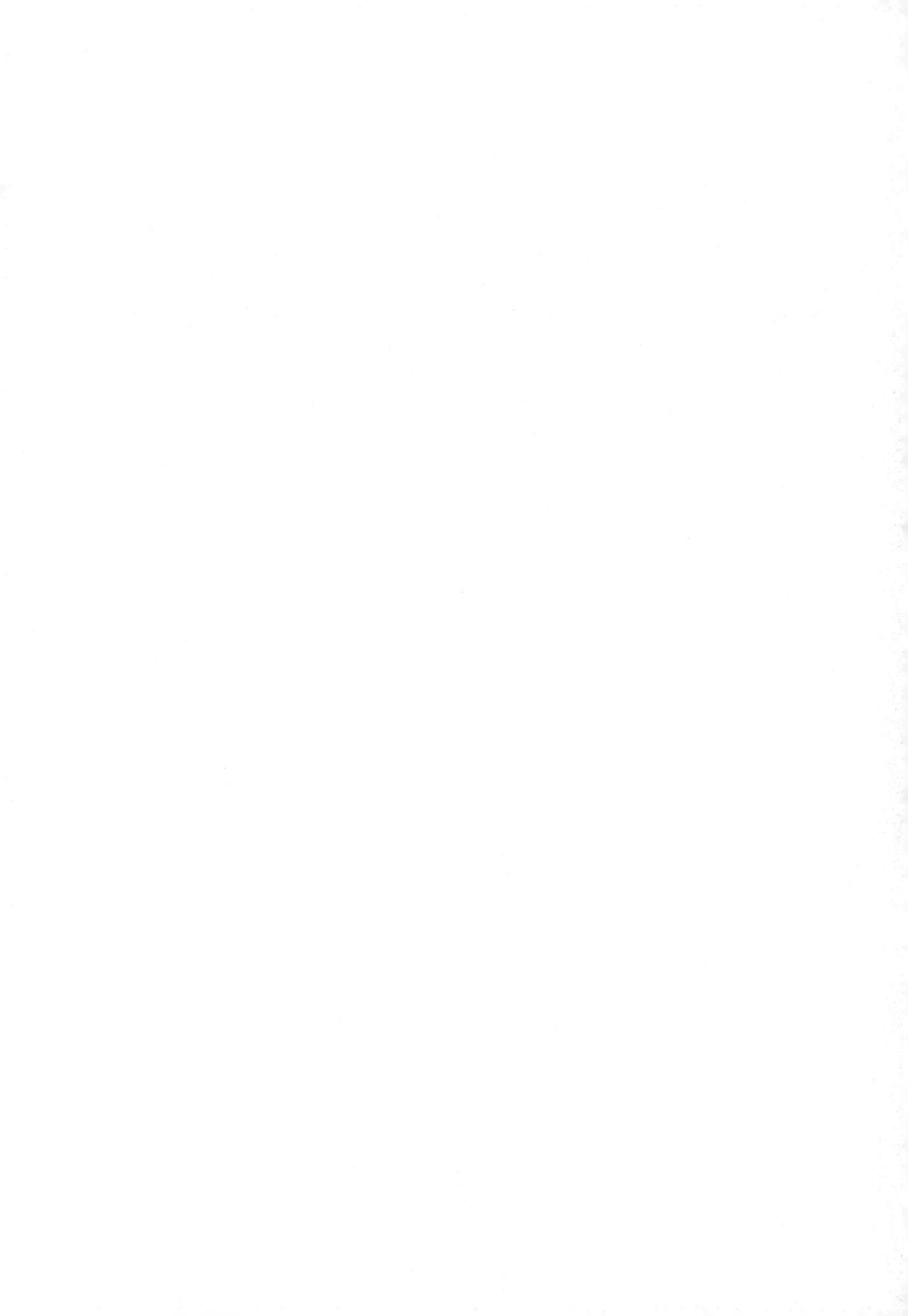

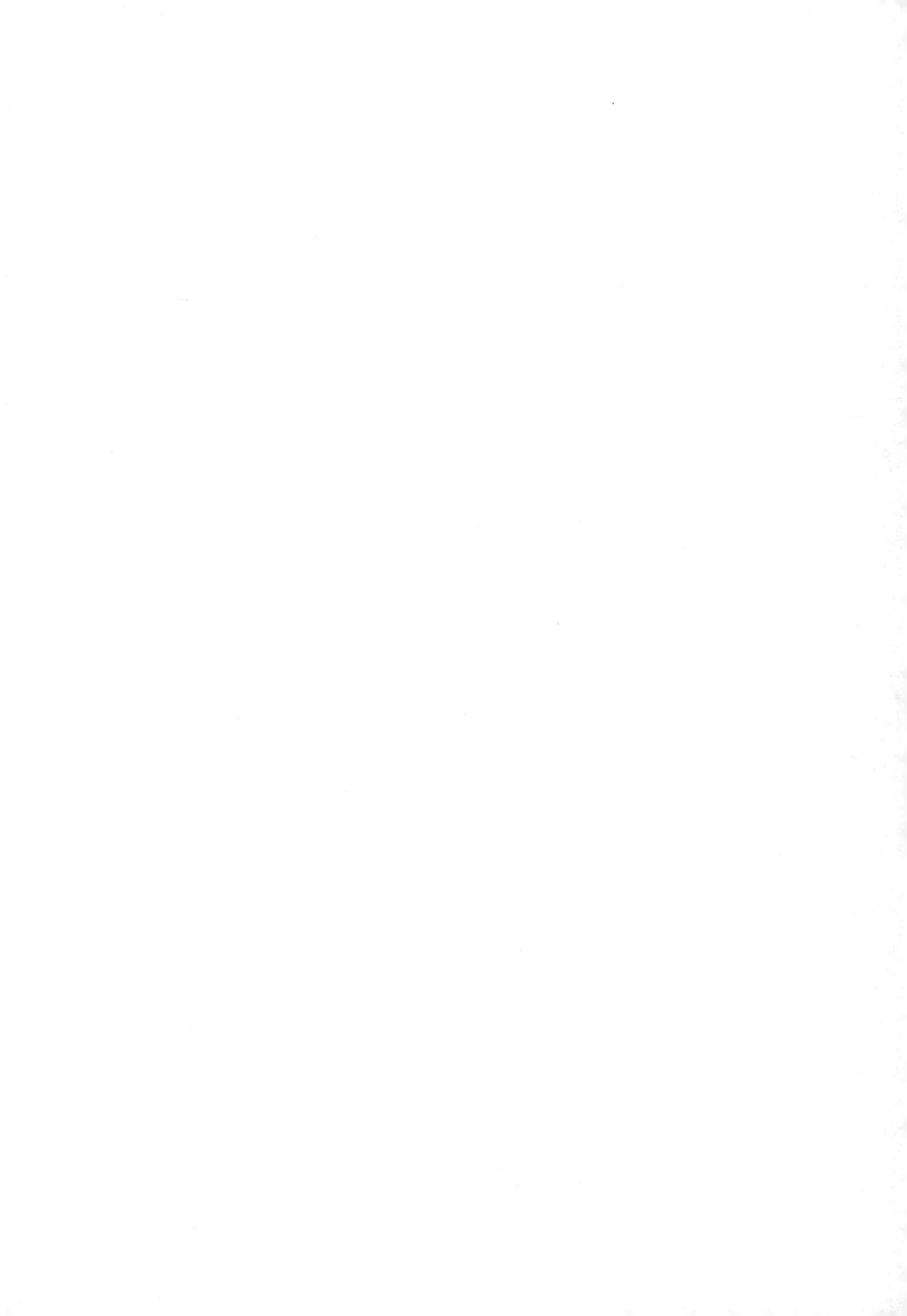

Printed in Great Britain
by Amazon